*Comments on* **Eczema and your child: a parent's guide**
*from readers*

'The tone of the book is very sensible and considered. It addresses the sorts of questions we are asked all the time.'

*Mercy Jeyasingham,*
*Director of Education and Training, National Eczema Society*

'I enjoyed reading this book and I think it fulfills a very useful purpose. It gets down to the "nitty-gritty" of atopic eczema management and addresses the questions that are most frequently asked in a clinic setting. If only there were time to answer them. The book is well written and authoritative.'

*Dr Mary Judge,*
*Consultant Dermatologist, Royal Bolton Hospital*

# A PARENT'S GUIDE

# ECZEMA
## and your child

**Tim Mitchell** MBCHB, DRCOG, DPD
*General Practitioner and Clinical Assistant in
Dermatology; Founder member of the Primary Care
Dermatology Society; and Specialist Adviser to the All Party
Parliamentary Group on Skin*

**David Paige** MBBS, MA, MRCP
*Consultant Dermatologist at The Royal London Hospital,
Queen Elizabeth Hospital for Children, Hackney, London,
and St Bartholomew's Hospital, London*

**Karen Spowart** RSCN, RGN
*Clinical Nurse Specialist, Paediatric Dermatology, Queen
Elizabeth Hospital for Children, Hackney, London*

CLASS PUBLISHING · LONDON

Printing history
First published 1998

The authors and publishers welcome feedback from the users of this book. Please contact the publishers.
**Class Publishing (London) Ltd, Barb House, Barb Mews,
London W6 7PA
Telephone: 0171 371 2119
Fax: 0171 371 2878 [International +44171]**

A CIP catalogue record for this book is available from the British Library

ISBN 1 872362 86 9

Designed by Wendy Bann

Edited by Gillian Clarke

Index by Valerie Elliston

Cartoons by Jane Taylor

Produced by Landmark Production Consultants Ltd, Princes Risborough

Typesetting by DP Photosetting, Aylesbury, Bucks

Printed and bound in Great Britain by Clays Ltd, St Ives plc

# Contents

# Acknowledgements

We are grateful to all the people who have helped in the production of this book, and in particular we thank the following for their contributions and support:

Leigh Mitchell for her skill in deciphering handwriting and producing the original typescript;

Mercy Jeyasingham of the National Eczema Society for her help and advice, and for reviewing the final draft;

the staff of the National Eczema Society for collecting most of the questions;

Mary Judge, Consultant Dermatologist in Manchester, for reviewing the final draft;

and last, but certainly not least, the children and their parents who asked the questions and contributed to the section on 'My child's eczema'. Many of them wished to remain anonymous, and we have respected this by changing their names.

# Foreword
## by Dr Martin M. Black

President of the British Association of Dermatologists

Atopic eczema (or childhood eczema, infantile eczema, atopic dermatitis) is one of the most common forms of eczema in childhood. It has a prevalence of 5–20% by the age of 11 years in children in temperate developed countries such as the UK. In our multicultural society all ethnic groups can be affected, but the disease may be even more prevalent in African/Caribbean or Asian children living here. Atopic eczema is more common in children than in adults and, like asthma, the prevalence seems to be slowly rising. Unlike asthma, however, atopic eczema does not have such a high profile with the general public or the media. The British Association of Dermatologists has for some time been keen to improve the management and care of eczema sufferers and has a close liaison with the National Eczema Society in this endeavour. Recently the Association promoted the first National Audit of atopic eczema management in secondary care, the results of which will be published shortly.

There is still a good deal of ignorance about eczema, and *Eczema and your child* does much to inform about all aspects of eczema. The three authors – a consultant dermatologist (Dr David Paige), a GP with a long-standing special interest in dermatology (Dr Tim Mitchell) and a clinical nurse specialist in paediatric dermatology (Mrs Karen Spowart) – are ideally suited to contribute to the book. Their involvement and important contributions to it stress the importance of teamwork in the management of eczema, because each role is vital to a successful outcome.

The text is very practical and user friendly. In a systematic series of chapters the authors endeavour to answer a series of questions about eczema from anxious parents. These are all relevant questions, which can at various times be asked during skin consultations. At present, specialist dermatology services are under great pressure and there may not be sufficient time to answer all parents' concerns. This book goes a very long way to helping everyone to understand eczema better.

I learned a good deal of practical tips from reading the book and I know that you will also. Let us all try to be better informed and active in promoting the welfare and future for eczema sufferers everywhere.

# Foreword
## by Peter Lapsley

Chief Executive, the National Eczema Society

The National Eczema Society welcomes the publication of *Eczema and your child: a parent's guide*.

Eczema knows no age barriers but is especially common in children, affecting between 5 and 15% of them. Although it varies enormously in severity, it almost always causes dryness, cracking and splitting of the skin and an inflamed rash that itches intensely. The desire to scratch can be irresistible. Scratching damages the skin further and can lead to weeping, bleeding and infection.

It is not only the child with eczema who is affected by it. At home, loss of sleep, time spent on treatment and dressings, and the need to modify the home environment can disrupt family life severely. School can present children with their first experience of prejudice, teasing and bullying, exposing them to a new range of potential irritants and difficulty in managing their eczema with no parent around to help.

*Eczema and your child* provides answers to many of the questions parents ask about such issues and to others as well. Written by three highly respected dermatology professionals, in collaboration with the National Eczema Society, it is both authoritative and readable. We commend it most warmly.

# The Charter for People for Eczema

In common with all patients, people with eczema need:
- Respect for their well-being, dignity, individual needs and privacy; also for their personal wishes concerning the relief of pain or termination of treatment.
- Safety through adequate staffing, well-maintained premises and equipment, proper investment in training and research, and thorough vetting of new drugs and medical procedures.
- Redress when things go wrong which is timely and appropriate and includes courteous explanations and apologies where necessary.

In particular, people with eczema need:
- Access to the full range of services when and where they are needed. Difficulties with language, costs, mobility or the long-term nature of eczema should not be a barrier to care.
- Full diagnosis and explanation of the type of eczema and its possible causes. Prognosis, including information on the possible impact on life-style, and demonstration and instructions on the appropriate use of medications and treatments, such as bandages.
- Respect for and recognition of the intellectual capacity, experience and knowledge of the patient and representative or carer. The nature and volatility of eczema are such that their observations should be fully taken into account by the medical team and used when decisions are made on improving and monitoring health care.
- Assurance of adequate primary health care resources to enable routine treatment to be conducted in the community rather than in hospital. The good of the patient should be considered a priority against costs in areas such as:
    receiving adequate supplies of medications, dressings and aids;
    adequate training for the primary health care team in teaching about the appropriate use of medications or bandages
- The right of choice to change GPs, have a second opinion, be consulted on treatment, hospital care or sex of doctor, or the

freedom to use complementary medicine, all without prejudice to continued support. The nature and state of knowledge and the multifactorial nature of eczema mean that a range of treatments and a policy of caring for and understanding of the whole person are important.

- Communication by health professionals in clear and comprehensible terms and adequate to the patient's needs. This could include options for treatment, clinical trials, likely outcomes, waiting times, complaints procedures and offer of access to the NES, its information, publications and support systems.
- Guidance on general or specific requirements in relation to lifestyle, education, employment and welfare benefits, recognising that ignorance about eczema in the community can result in misunderstanding, stigma and discrimination. Use of NES literature can help patients reach their full potential.
- Consistency, continuity and accountability of medical care through a clearly defined chain of command so that there is always a specified person or department who is responsible for an individual's care. The many causes of eczema and aspects of treatment make this of particular importance.
- Immediacy of consultation, recognising that eczema can flare to acute proportions in a matter of hours. The 'open appointment' system should be made available to all identified as needing this service.
- Communication between systems of medical care where a patient needs treatment from other specialties; e.g. when a person with eczema requires treatment for asthma or is in a surgical ward, or when a child with eczema is cared for in a paediatric ward.
- Confidentiality of medical records and entitlement of private examination if requested, recognising that eczema can be a disfiguring and potentially embarrassing condition.
- Continuing support, especially if the eczema becomes chronic and palliative care is required, together with care and support over periods of acute ill-health caused by the eczema.
- Consideration of family needs and the particularly disruptive nature of eczema, which can affect partners, carers and siblings. Their particular needs should be recognized as linked but separate from those of the person with eczema.

# Introduction

'Eczema' is a word applied to a number of different skin disorders, all of which give typical inflammation of the outer layer of the skin. **Atopic** eczema (see Glossary) is one of the most common skin diseases in childhood, so it is the major focus of this book. It is the type of eczema that is often associated with two other illnesses that also carry the label 'atopic' – asthma and hayfever. The three conditions have an inherited basis and so tend to run in families.

The incidence of atopic eczema seems to have increased over the last 30 years, and it is now estimated that 5–15% of children in developed countries will have the disease at some stage in their childhood. Trying to count the cost of this may help make sense of the statistics. The annual financial cost of atopic eczema in the UK is over £450 million and the 'emotional cost' – the impact it has on the lives of affected children and their families – is even greater but impossible to quantify. We live in a very image-conscious society, so visible skin disease attracts attention – often generating hostility and rejection rather than sympathy. We have heard mothers complain that total strangers have come up to them in the street and accused them of scalding their child or of neglect. Young children have complained of bullying at school and of classmates refusing to sit next to them. There is, unfortunately, a lot of ignorance about skin diseases in general.

Childhood atopic eczema varies enormously in severity.

It can be a mild condition causing no more than occasional irritation and inconvenience or, more rarely, it can be a very severe disorder with profound effects on a child's growth, education and social development. In these severe cases, eczema should be seen as a 'family disorder', because all family members can have their lives disrupted by a child's illness. Fortunately, most children have eczema of a less severe nature and, as long as appropriate advice and information about the disease is made available to parents, they should be able to manage and control the condition rather than having the eczema controlling them. This should allow the affected child to have a relatively normal childhood with minimal disruption from the eczema.

It is very easy to say this and we are aware of how difficult it can be to obtain such advice and to feel confident about putting it into practice. In our experience, most parents have received conflicting information about eczema from a number of different sources. Everybody seems to have an opinion about eczema – its causes and its treatments. One father said that he felt more people had an

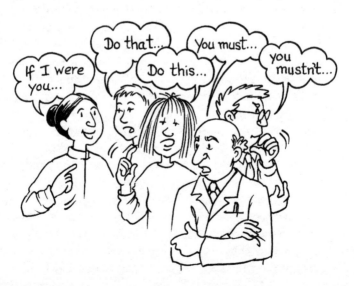

opinion about eczema than about who should be picked for the England football team! For example:

the neighbour says 'you mustn't bath your child more than once a week';
the health visitor says 'you must bath your child every day';

the GP says 'weak topical steroids are safe';
the pharmacist says 'weak topical steroids cause skin thinning';

the specialist says 'use this steroid on the face';
the packaging on the steroid says 'do not use on the face'.

The information provided by the manufacturer can also say 'do not use on broken skin' and/or 'use sparingly'.

**You are confused!**

You feel that all eczema looks like 'broken skin' and what does 'sparingly' mean? You may well ask why there are so many seemingly contradictory opinions about this skin disorder, and there may be a number of explanations.

- There is no single correct treatment for eczema. Many different treatment approaches may produce the same outcome and all may be equally worthwhile. Wherever possible, therapy should be tailored to the wishes of the individual child and his or her parents.
- What works for one child may not work for another, even in the same family.
- The most important aspect of eczema treatment relies on the application of creams or ointments to the skin yet scant regard is paid to instructions on how to apply these, how frequently and in what quantities. If these issues are not adequately explained or demonstrated, treatment will not be used correctly and will lead to apparent 'treatment failure' even when the therapy is appropriate.

- The natural history of eczema is that it will get better and get worse regardless of therapy. In most instances we can't explain why this happens but there is a tendency to look at the events preceding any such change (e.g. diet, new herbal therapy, change in the weather) and see these as the cause.
- We are sorry to say that the lack of dermatology training among people in the medical and allied professions does not help to improve their understanding of conditions such as atopic eczema. Many of the parents and children we spoke to when preparing this book were unhappy about treatment given by their GP. This is a common problem and the training of doctors needs to be changed before the situation will dramatically improve. Eczema can make up as much as 5% of a GP's workload yet it is possible to become a GP without any formal training in dealing with skin disease. There are a great many GPs who are very good at treating eczema but this is usually because they have taken the time, trouble and often expense to learn a lot more about it.
- There is even confusion over the definition of the word 'eczema'. This is made worse by the fact that some people use the term 'dermatitis'. In many ways these two words mean the same thing but people (especially doctors) often speak of dermatitis when referring to eczema caused by external factors, especially at work. We must remember there are **different types of eczema**, and these have different causes and different approaches to treatment.

We will try to lead you through the maze of fact and fiction concerning eczema, its causes and its management. We will concentrate on atopic eczema because this is responsible for most of the problems encountered with childhood eczema. We freely acknowledge that we do not have all the answers but we will try to provide a sensible approach based on our experience in dealing with affected families. We do not claim that this is the only valid approach but we hope it will prove educational and of practical use in your day-to-day management of this common skin disorder.

To finish on an optimistic note, you should keep in mind that eczema can usually be treated effectively and that most children with eczema will eventually improve spontaneously as they grow older.

## HOW TO USE THIS BOOK

Every parent reading this book will have a different need for information, so it is arranged to help you. You do not have to read it straight through but can dip in and out of different sections. The questions are arranged into chapters and sections, with cross-referencing to allow you to follow a topic through different parts of the book. Some repetition is inevitable but this is usually important information that is worth repeating.

The first part of the book covers what is known about what causes (and what doesn't cause) eczema, with discussion about the different patterns and possible implications. The central part deals with treatment and the final part deals with the vital areas of how it affects both your life and your child's life. To **manage** eczema, as opposed to just **treating** it, the social issues and psychological effects are just as important.

Not everyone will agree with every answer we give but argument and discussion are essential in medicine to help us move forward in our understanding of any disease. You can help us improve by letting us have your comments both about the answers and any questions you may have that are not answered. Please write to us:

c/o Class Publishing (London) Ltd
Barb House
Barb Mews
LONDON W6 7PA

# My child's eczema

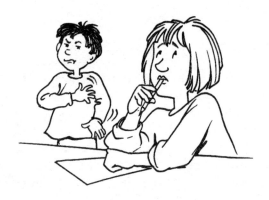

**Tony, now 30 years old, looks back on his childhood**

It was a bit of a pain having eczema when I was growing up. It was the itching that was the worst thing. An intense drive to rub, scratch or even tear at my skin. Anything to relieve that sensation – so difficult to describe – of irritating tickling beneath the skin. Worse than falling over or grazing your knee, perhaps, because I knew that, unlike most pains, the itch would return. And it doesn't help when parents ask you not to scratch. Although I wanted to follow my parents' advice, when it came to choosing between duty to parents and relieving the itch, the itch won, hands down, every time. When you've scratched the spot it is a wonderful relief as well – until you remember that the relief is only temporary and until you realise the damage done to your skin.

Summer could be the worst time. Long sticky car journeys, after which the backs of my knees would stick to the seat leather. And I just knew that a visit to Gran with her cats, or some dumb relative with dogs and no end of other furry things, would bring me out in a rash all over, and make my nose and eyes run to boot.

Yet swimming, running around and having fun were always possible. I always knew that there were plenty of other children with eczema and asthma, both at school and where I lived. I learned to control the eczema, to know what made it worse or better, and which ointments and moisturisers to use. And if there was an acute flare-up of my eczema – which there always was every now and again – I learned how to deal with it.

## From Stuart's parents

Lee, our first baby, was diagnosed as having infantile eczema. So when Stuart arrived and had skin like peaches and cream we were delighted. By the time Stuart was six months old, though, he also started to develop patchy dry skin, and by the time he was 18 months he had had his first hospital admission for chronic atopic eczema. He was in hospital for two weeks and was being bathed twice daily and creamed, and then having Ichthopaste (zinc oxide and ichthammol paste) and Coban (cohesive) bandages applied almost everywhere. Over the years we got used to having to do this daily routine, and to Stuart it was a way of life. It affected him at school, as you can imagine; children can be very cruel and this sometimes resulted in Stuart not wanting to go to school.

As he grew up and reached the age of nine years the eczema seemed to more or less disappear, but as soon as Stuart reached puberty, unfortunately, the eczema came back and resulted in his having to be admitted to hospital again. His eczema can make him feel really miserable and moody. He still says to us 'Why can't I have skin like normal people?' but we tell him that he **is** normal – it is just unfortunate he has a skin condition and that, hopefully, some day it will resolve. Stuart has had four hospital admissions, after which the eczema does clear; but, because of stresses from school and studying for GCSE exams, the condition seems to worsen. As a family we have always supported him and put Stuart's eczema down to a way of life for us all, in the hope that one day he will grow out of this condition for good.

## Stuart (aged 15)

I have had eczema since I was six months old, so I've never really known any different. As a small child I had to have two baths a day and be wrapped in bandages all over. I was on a special diet for years, and I still have to watch what I eat and drink. It didn't affect me at school when I was younger, but as I got older the other children's jibes got worse. It sometimes affected my schooling because, when my eczema became infected, I couldn't go to school. Over all the years of using steroid creams and strong steroid tablets, I have developed cataracts in both eyes, which will need to be operated on.

I'm now taking my GCSE exams at school and hope that, once I have taken them and, hopefully, passed, my eczema will go, because stress has a big part to play with this complaint. I've been in hospital for the fourth time and am taking new medication (cyclosporin) that is working – hopefully, for good.

## From Brett's mother

We adopted Brett when he was four months old, and it was often remarked upon how white and unusual his skin looked. It was not until he was eight months old that we noticed dry rings appearing around by his ankles; when he was one year old, sores started appearing on his wrists. We consulted our GP and we were told that it was infantile eczema, given some creams and medication, and advised that, after a while, it would clear up.

Unfortunately, it did not clear up. During the next six months, after frequent visits to our GP, Brett was admitted to hospital because the whole of his body had become infected and needed intensive treatment that could not be carried out at home. Since then, Brett has been in hospital twice more because of the severity of the eczema and when it has become infected.

Brett is now six years old and for the last five and half years it has been a constant vigil to check that he does not scratch, and to find ways to keep him occupied so that he does not think about the irritation that his skin is causing him. We also have to 'cream' him several times every day – which he doesn't like, so applying the cream will often be a battle of wills. Bandages also have to be used most weeks, which again Brett finds uncomfortable and restricting. This is because the bandages have to be put over his fingers, so they act like mittens.

The effect this has had on our family life has been to cause us many a sleepless night because of Brett's scratching, making his skin sore. He will wake up crying and when we go in to see to him his skin will be raw and bleeding from the scratching; so in the middle of the night we will have to cream him down again and reapply the bandages, which Brett finds quite distressing.

I also have to keep his bed and room immaculately clean and free from house dust mite which gets into the bedding, as we have found that this irritates Brett's condition and causes even more problems.

We have found that Brett's having this condition seems to dominate our life-style, as we are constantly having to watch him and make time for the special care of bathing him and applying his creams. Also, if we go away from home for any time, we have to take all his medication, creams, bath oils and bandages with us.

As well as all this there is the emotional side of the condition. We often find it distressing when trying to stop Brett from scratching; he will get irritable and upset, and we feel there is nothing we can do to relieve his suffering.

## John's mother

Looking back over my experience of dealing with a child with eczema, a wide range of emotions spring to mind. Besides its being a relentless and difficult task, the feeling of hopelessness was predominant. I could never seem to make it stop for him. I will never forget coming back in the car from a particularly difficult holiday abroad with him and turning round to find that he had scratched his arms so much that they were bleeding quite a lot. The shock of it was quite numbing. I am now at a stage where I can try to talk to him about the scratching, and he understands that his creams help him – to the extent that he will ask for cream if something is hurting.

## Sophie's mother

Sophie developed eczema aged about three months. I suppose I shouldn't have been surprised, because her father had terrible eczema as a child and continued to have mild eczema as an adult, and I have mild asthma. My first reaction was guilt for breast-feeding her for only three months, because I went back to work. My next thought was relief that it didn't involve her face.

Her father regaled us all with stories of his mother wrapping him in a pillow case to stop him scratching at night, and her embarrassment at the stares he would receive, with his face red, scratched and bleeding, whenever she took him out in the pram. I was complacent, convinced that the ugly red patches on the back of Sophie's knees, her elbows and her wrists would all disappear by the time she was two. But they didn't. Her eczema got worse, affecting particularly her hands. Our GP prescribed oilatum to put in the bath, aqueous cream as an emollient and to use instead of soap, and 1% hydrocortisone. This improved things but as soon as we stopped the steroid cream the eczema flared again. A locum GP refused to give me a repeat prescription of 1% hydrocortisone and told me that most eczema in children of this age was due to an allergy to milk and dairy products. The guilt I felt about introducing cow's milk too early resurfaced. We tried soya products for two days – yuk!

We tried to teach Sophie to remember to put cream on her hands and the itchy bits after her bath in the mornings and evenings. We established a routine, but even now (she is seven) we are often to be heard nagging her – but we do not want to give her the impression that, if her eczema gets worse, it is her fault. She finds it hard to understand why she has eczema and her three younger sisters do not. Strangers or friends and family who held her hands would often flinch, look at her hands to try to understand why they felt so dry and rough. A friend has advised me that Sophie may need a stronger steroid for her hands, but our GP will give only 1% hydrocortisone.

Sophie's hands are now much better, as are her wrists, but her knees and the backs of her thighs have got worse. I have stopped trying to explain the changes that happen at different times and that some parts of the body will be affected more than others. I remain confident that things will improve as she gets older, as they did in her father. She is learning to live with eczema and will now ask for some topical steroid if she is itching. She has learned that pinching to inflict mild pain relieves the itch and will ask us to do this sometimes. She often scratches at night, but fortunately rarely wakes herself up.

It is still a struggle to get topical steroids from the GP and this problem is made worse by Sophie's father 'stealing' bits of her hydrocortisone to use on his fingers when he has forgotten to wear gloves for the washing up. His rapid reaction to detergent reminds us both that, although he has grown out of severe eczema (and hopefully, therefore, Sophie will too), he must always remain vigilant.

# CHAPTER 1

## *What is eczema?*

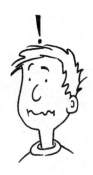

'Eczema' is a Greek word meaning 'to boil or flow out', and anyone who has had acute eczema will understand how appropriate this is. Acute (short-term) inflammation can cause the skin to blister and weep against a background redness and an intense feeling of itch. Eczema is, however, often chronic (long-term) without the wetness and the skin tends to be dry, flaky and thickened.

## DIFFERENT TYPES OF ECZEMA

Eczema is not a specific diagnosis but simply a way that the skin can behave; there are different types and varying causes. The main types of eczema seen in childhood are:

- atopic eczema,
- seborrhoeic eczema.

11

Less common are:

- irritant eczema,
- contact (or allergic) eczema,
- pompholyx eczema of the hands and feet.

## Is eczema the same as dermatitis?

Yes, these two words are effectively the same and it is annoying that they confuse people. The Americans tend to use the word dermatitis more commonly. Also some people use the word dermatitis to imply that the rash is due to an external or occupational cause. Whichever word you prefer to use, it is best to qualify it with a preceding word such as atopic, seborrhoeic or contact. Pharmacists have recently been allowed to sell some treatments for 'dermatitis' rather than 'eczema', which also adds to the confusion.

## What is pompholyx?

'Pompholyx' is a word used to describe a pattern of eczema affecting the hands or feet, which typically shows blistering and is usually very itchy. It comes in recurrent attacks, which may last for some weeks. The blisters often run along the sides of the fingers. Pompholyx eczema is more common in hot weather and can occur in three types:

- atopic eczema;
- in isolation (the cause here is unknown);
- contact (allergic) eczema (this is very rare in children).

## My baby has bad nappy rash despite regular changing of nappies and using a barrier cream. Could she have eczema affecting the nappy area?

There are actually three types of eczema that can affect the nappy area. The most common is irritant eczema (nappy rash), which affects nearly all children to some degree. This simply reflects that urine and faeces are irritant to the skin if left in contact for prolonged periods. This type of nappy rash usually spares the skin in the groin. The skin fold between the leg and tummy looks normal but is surrounded on either side by red, inflamed skin.

As you are already doing all the right things to prevent nappy rash, your baby may have one of the other types of eczema (atopic or seborrhoeic). Both these tend to involve rather than spare the skin fold at the top of the leg. Atopic eczema is normally very itchy and you may see eczema in the skin folds elsewhere on the body (e.g. in front of the elbows or behind the knees). In contrast, seborrhoeic eczema tends not to be itchy. It may be associated with scaling in the scalp (cradle cap) and greasy, yellowish scales.

**The health visitor says my baby has cradle cap and that this is a type of eczema. Is this true?**

Yes, this is a type of eczema called seborrhoeic eczema. It is very common in the first few months of life but very rare during later childhood. It presents with scaling in the scalp (cradle cap) and sometimes a greasy, scaly rash elsewhere on the body, especially in the nappy area. Despite an often extensive rash, your baby is not usually itchy and will probably not be distressed by it. It should resolve spontaneously within the first few months of life but, because of its appearance, you might prefer to seek treatment from your GP.

**I get very confused by all the different types of eczema that can affect the skin. You say that the final process in the skin is the same for all of them. Why can't we just call it all eczema and get on with treating it?**

Despite the fact that, at microscopic level, the skin looks very similar for the different types of eczema, this just reflects the final event, as the skin can only behave in so many ways when disordered. However, the main reason for trying to label the disorders accurately is that the cause, severity and outcome vary enormously between the different eczemas. Whilst some of the treatments are similar for the different types of eczema, there are many that are more specific so **accurate diagnosis is essential**.

## WHAT HAPPENS IN THE SKIN?

**What happens in the skin of people with eczema?**

To explain what happens you need to understand the structure of the skin as seen down a microscope. The skin consists of three layers.

- The outer layer is called the **epidermis**. This contains a 'brick wall' of skin cells (keratinocytes) that are held together by a 'cement' mostly made up of fats or lipids. The skin cells constantly reproduce to replace the daily shedding of dead cells from the surface. The lipid cement acts as a barrier against the environment. It prevents the skin losing too much water and prevents noxious (poisonous) substances getting in.
- The middle layer of skin is called the **dermis**. This consists of tough structural fibres called collagen and elastin, which provide strength and elasticity to the skin. It also contains blood vessels that supply nutrients and oxygen to both the dermis and the epidermis.
- The deepest layer of skin is called the **subcutaneous layer**, and is made up predominantly of an insulating layer of fat.

In eczema it is the **dermis** and **epidermis** that are affected. The epidermis shows the most marked changes. The inflammation leads to leaky blood vessels and fluid collects between the keratinocytes, causing them to separate. The brick wall takes on a sponge-like appearance. The constant rubbing/scratching with eczema causes the epidermis to regenerate more quickly, and so it becomes thickened.

Finally, eczema causes changes in the upper part of the dermis. This region becomes flooded with white blood cells, which are part of the body's immune system or defences. They leak out of the vessels and even pass up into the epidermis. Current evidence suggests that it is these cells that drive the whole process of inflammation in the skin.

**Why does my son's skin weep fluid and feel wet?**

If you think of the epidermis changing to look like a sponge, you can imagine the fluid leaking out and causing blisters that break easily to give a wet weeping area.

**Why is skin with eczema so susceptible to irritants?**

As fluid accumulates in the epidermis, the 'bricks' separate and the 'cement' becomes disrupted. This makes the skin barrier less effective, allowing the irritants through to the more sensitive dermis. Some irritants, such as soaps, work by dissolving the lipid 'cement', leading to further breakdown of the skin's barrier function.

**How does our doctor know that my child has eczema?**

As there are no specific tests for most types of eczema, your doctor will have reached a diagnosis on what we call 'clinical grounds'. This means taking a careful history of the problem and any family history of eczema, asthma or hayfever. Examination of the skin will add to the clues in the history, allowing a diagnosis to be made.

Some children with atopic eczema may have abnormal blood tests, such as high levels of an antibody called immunoglobulin E (IgE). Antibodies are chemicals made by the body as a defence against infection. Children may also show high IgE levels to specific allergens (the causes or triggers of allergy), which can be measured by a blood test called an ELISA test (this is discussed further under allergy testing, a little later). However, these tests do not diagnose atopic eczema. You can have abnormal blood tests and never develop eczema. Furthermore, you may develop eczema despite having normal levels of IgE antibody. So your child will be pleased to hear that blood tests are not a routine part of diagnosing eczema.

**My 6-year-old son has developed very bad eczema since starting school. Why is this?**

There may be a number of explanations, depending on his previous history and any family history.

Irritant eczema is one possibility as this often affects the hands – which get more wear and tear than other parts of the body. This can be seen in children who repeatedly expose their skin to irritants such as soaps, detergents, paints, sandpits and so forth, and this of course happens at school. It is important to teach children to wash their hands but some may do this rather too often and damage the skin. Strong irritants used frequently can give anybody eczema.

Irritant eczema is more likely to occur if your son has pre-existing atopic eczema, in which the skin's barrier will already be damaged to some degree; this means that some children will actually have two types of eczema.

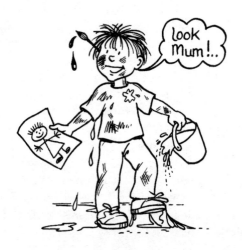

Finally, contact (allergic) eczema is a possibility but it is much rarer in children than in adults. This may be because it often takes years of repeated exposure to certain substances (e.g. nickel, rubber or perfume) before they cause an allergy. The eczema is usually localised to areas of skin that have come into contact with the offending agent. Rubber gloves can cause contact eczema of the hands but these are rarely worn by children. The history and the distribution of the eczema normally arouse one's suspicions. Contact eczema can be confirmed or ruled out by a specific test called 'patch testing', carried out by the hospital dermatology department. The test involves having little aluminium discs, each with a small amount of a suspect substance (allergen) taped onto the back for three days. Any reactions are noted at that stage and checked again after a further two days. (See also the section on testing, a few pages further on.)

**My family are from India and I have noticed that my child's eczema looks different from eczema in white children. Why is this?**

I am afraid we cannot explain why there are different patterns of eczema in different racial groups but you are absolutely right to have spotted the difference. Eczema often affects the flexures (the creases in front of the elbows and behind the knees) but, in Asian and particularly in African/Caribbean children, eczema sometimes shows a reverse pattern, affecting the extensor surfaces (behind the elbows and in front of the knees). There may be other differences in children with more pigmented skin.

In African/Caribbean and Asian children eczema is more likely to produce:

- thickening of the skin (lichenification),
- lumpy or papular skin (papular or follicular eczema),
- a marked increase or decrease in pigmentation of the skin after the eczema has settled down.

# WHY DOES IT ITCH?

**Why does skin itch with eczema?**

Surprisingly, this is a very difficult question to answer as the current scientific understanding of itch is really very poor. We do know that certain small nerve fibres in the skin transmit 'itch' signals to the spinal cord and then to the brain. These same fibres can also transmit pain signals. There are certain centres in the brain that receive these signals and then interpret them either as an itch sensation or, sometimes, as pain. Why people with eczema itch simply isn't known. It may be that the dry inflamed skin of eczema somehow fires off these nerve fibres, causing itch. However, there is also some evidence to suggest that these skin nerve fibres and the chemical signals (neurotransmitters) that they contain may be abnormal in eczema, and it may be that the skin changes are 'secondary' – i.e. that they are the result of the damage done by scratching. A lot more research needs to be done into the mechanisms of itch before we have a clearer picture.

# FACTS AND FIGURES

**How many children are affected by eczema?**

Current estimates suggest that somewhere between 5% and 15% of children in developed countries will develop eczema.

**Do more boys get eczema than girls?**

Yes, atopic eczema is somewhat more common in boys than in girls.

**Two other children in my son's class have eczema. Is eczema becoming more common?**

Yes, indeed it is. Over the last 40 years eczema has shown a two- to five-fold increase, depending on which studies you believe. Certainly all studies agree that eczema is increasing even if they don't agree by how much.

### Is my child with eczema likely to still have it when he grows up?

Most children (more than 90%) with early-onset eczema (it starts when they are less than one year old) will grow out of it before adult life. However, if your child developed eczema for the first time late on in childhood, the chances of improvement are less.

About 5–10% of children with atopic eczema will develop hand eczema in adult life even if they have **grown out** of their original eczema. This is especially true if they take up certain careers (e.g. as a hairdresser, mechanic or nurse) that cause repeated irritation and damage to the hands.

### My baby has eczema; is he likely to get asthma as well?

Eczema, asthma and hayfever tend to go together, as mentioned in the Introduction. Asthma is itself a common disease and can affect up to 10% of all people at some point in their lives. Your baby will have an increased risk of getting asthma at some stage – perhaps as high as 50%. Eczema tends to come on earlier in life than asthma, and there is research going on to see if the likelihood of developing asthma can be lessened. You should discuss things further with your family doctor.

### How can I tell if my child is getting asthma?

If your child has a persistent wheeze or is coughing at night, asthma might be the cause and you should discuss this with your doctor.

**I moved to England from Jamaica 16 years ago. Two of my children have eczema and I have other friends who also have affected children. Is eczema more common in the UK than in the West Indies?**

Yes, it seems that eczema is much more common in the UK. A recent study showed that eczema is almost twice as common among school children in London than in Kingston, Jamaica. When looking only at black children, it was present in up to four times more children in London than in Kingston. We also feel that this increased incidence may be seen in children from India and Bangladesh.

**I had bad eczema as a child. What is the likelihood of any of my children developing eczema?**

There is certainly an increased risk of your child's developing eczema but this is difficult to quantify exactly. The risk is about 20–30%. If both you and your husband have had atopic eczema, the risk would exceed 50%. However, severity doesn't run true; i.e. even if you had bad eczema, your child may have mild eczema and, unfortunately, vice versa.

# CHAPTER 2

## What causes eczema?

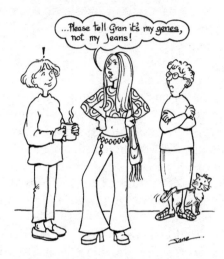

It must be so frustrating for parents who want to know why their child has eczema, as this simple question is beyond our knowledge to answer completely. We will try to explain what our current understanding is and also try to dispel some of the myths and establish what does **not** cause eczema. It seems inevitable that myths and untruths arise when we don't fully understand the causes of eczema but, sadly, those misconceptions can lead to wholly inappropriate treatment and inadequately controlled disease. If there were a simple answer to 'What causes eczema?', you would not be reading this book!

## INHERITANCE AND ALLERGY

want to find out exactly what is causing my son's eczema. How can I get him tested?

You have asked one of the most difficult questions to

answer because we don't have a complete understanding o
the cause(s) of atopic eczema. Some people think that it is al
due to a single allergy and that avoidance of the allergei
(the cause or trigger of the allergy) will result in a cure. Thi
may apply to a rare type of childhood eczema called contac
(or allergic) eczema but unfortunately it is not that simple ii
atopic eczema.

We do know that there is a strong inherited or geneti
component to atopic eczema. If your son has inherited ;
certain gene, or combination of genes, this predisposes hin
to being 'atopic'. To date, three genes have been identifiec
that show a link with atopic disease, but it seems likely tha
there are other, as yet unidentified, genes that are importan
and we hope that some of these will be discovered over th
next few years. We do not yet understand the function o
these genes and we do not know which ones predispose t
eczema, asthma or hayfever – the three atopic diseases. It i
likely that various different gene combinations can lead t
atopic eczema, as this would explain why different trigger
are important in different patients and why eczema ha
more than one 'cause'.

In other words, if your son has a susceptibility to develo
eczema by having a particular group of genes, it may b
triggered by several different factors. Despite a lot c
research, the evidence for any one trigger is very limitec
and trials excluding or limiting exposure to differer
environmental factors (e.g. pets, woollen clothing, dust, ca
pollution) have been very disappointing in terms c
improving eczema. There is therefore no simple way to ge
your son tested and it is more likely that simple detectiv
work, looking at when it gets worse, may give you more of
clue. (For more about testing, though, see the section 'Ar
there any tests?' later in this chapter.)

## But isn't eczema caused by an allergy to something?

It depends what you mean by 'allergy'. The strictly scientif definition of allergy is 'when a substance causes an abnormally excessive response from the body's immune or defence system'. This may be measured by determining the levels of antibody in the blood or by showing a response by the body's white blood cells (lymphocytes). The allergic reaction should be reproducible by 'rechallenging' with the same substance – the same reaction is produced each time the substance is used.

However, many people use the word 'allergy' in a different way. They may use it to imply that a certain disorder is caused by a specific substance and that this disorder will disappear if the offending agent is avoided. Unfortunately, this is not the case with atopic eczema. It is perhaps best imagined as a built-in reaction that can be modified (but not caused) by the environment. Many things in the environment can make eczema worse (e.g. woollen clothes or dog

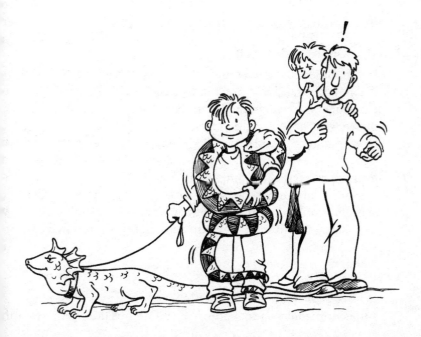

hair) but this may be purely as an irritant rather than as a true allergen.

**What type of dog can I have that will not irritate my son's eczema?**

Dogs, and indeed any animals with furry or hairy coats (e.g. horses, cats), shed their hair and skin into the environment. These small particles are made up of proteins that are 'foreign' to humans. They can irritate the skin without an allergic reaction taking place, especially if the skin is already damaged with eczema. They may also cause a genuine allergic response. Although breeds of dogs with shorter coats may spread their proteins around the house in lesser amounts, these will still be present in a significant quantity. All dogs therefore have the potential to make eczema worse, so it is probably best not to get a dog or other pet with a furry or hairy coat.

# ARE HOUSE DUST MITES INVOLVED?

**What are house dust mites?**

House dust mites are very small insects that are invisible to the naked eye. They are found in all of our homes and particularly like living in soft furnishings such as sofas, mattresses, carpets and duvets, where they are found in large numbers. Modern living standards with central heating seem to encourage their growth, and in practice they are difficult to eradicate completely.

House dust mites do seem to be important in making asthma worse and, although their role in atopic eczema is less well established, they are worth taking seriously in some cases.

**How do I know if my son is allergic to the house dust mite?**

It is easy to find evidence of allergy to house dust mite by subjecting your son to skin-prick testing but the result may not be very useful. Many people with eczema will have a positive reaction to house dust mite – and to many other allergens that do not seem to make their eczema worse. Many children without eczema also have positive reactions to house dust mite. If you suspect that house dust mite may be important in your son's eczema, it may be best to try some avoidance measures (see later in Chapter 4) rather than have the test done. The test itself involves putting on the skin drops of liquid that either contains mite extract in saline (salt water) or is just saline on its own. The skin is then pricked with a needle through each drop and the skin's reaction tested. A strong reaction to mite extract compared to saline indicates a positive result.

# IS DIET IMPORTANT?

**During a recent bout of sickness and diarrhoea my daughter's eczema almost disappeared. She ate hardly anything during this time. Could this mean that her eczema is related to the food she eats?**

Unfortunately, this is not the likeliest explanation for the improvement in her eczema. Diet has not been shown to be a major factor in causing eczema, despite many people's view to the contrary. You have to remember that eczema fluctuates in severity all the time, often for reasons that we can't explain. It is always tempting to look at 'what happened the day before' as the cause of a flare-up or an improvement, and doctors are no different from you in wanting a simple explanation.

Any infection (including tummy upsets) can improve eczema or cause a flare-up, presumably due to the effect it can have on the body's immune system or the fact that having a high temperature may make the skin more itchy. It is equally likely that your daughter's sickness had no effect on her eczema but that it simply was improving spontaneously at that time.

**Could something in my son's diet be causing his eczema?**

Although you don't say how old your son is, the answer is probably not. Diet may be important in the initial triggering of eczema in infants with an inherited susceptibility but it seems to have little to do with keeping eczema going or triggering it in older children. It is true that many parents and, indeed, some doctors think that diet is very important in eczema but evidence from research studies over the last few years does not support this view. Life would be a lot easier if diet did have a major impact but we have to believe the evidence from these well-conducted studies. We have used special diets in the past but they are normally disappointing in terms of improving the eczema and are difficult to stick to especially for children of school age.

Our advice to you is that, if there is a clear history of your son's eczema always worsening after eating a certain food, it would be worth a three-month trial of excluding that food – after taking advice from a dietician. If there is no improvement in his eczema after three months, that food should be gradually re-introduced. It cannot be over-emphasised that all attempts at dietary manipulation should be under the control of a dietician to ensure that there is adequate calorie, protein, calcium and vitamin replacement. We have seen children with malnutrition and even rickets from unsupervised severe exclusion diets, and unfortunately they both still had bad eczema.

**Will altering my diet during breast-feeding stop my baby from developing eczema? What else can I do to avoid triggering the condition?**

Eczema is an inherited condition but it is also influenced by environmental factors. We do not understand why it develops at a certain age in any one individual. There are important trigger factors but little is known about them. It has been suggested that the early diet of a child, particularly the exposure to dairy products, might be important in triggering eczema.

There is scant evidence to support the idea that, if you changed to a diet free from milk and eggs during breast-feeding, it might provide some protection against your baby developing eczema, especially if both you and the baby's father have a history of the condition. This view is still controversial and we would not recommend such a diet routinely. It would certainly need to be done under the guidance of a dietician.

There is rather stronger evidence to show that breast-feeding itself (rather than bottle-feeding) may protect against or delay the development of eczema. Whilst not all studies have shown this apparent benefit, until the situation is clarified it seems sensible to encourage breast-feeding in all mothers who have had an atopic disorder. Breast-feeding has many other advantages anyway, so we would support the motto 'Breast is Best'.

There is nothing else that you can do at this stage and it is very important that you do not feel guilty if your baby does develop eczema. Much more research needs to be done into identifying trigger factors in atopic eczema, so there may be more advice to give in the future.

**I want to continue breast-feeding my baby, but the eczema on my nipples is making this very difficult. Have you any advice that could help?**

Breast-feeding with eczema on the nipple or areola tissue round it can be troublesome from time to time, because this area can easily become infected with thrush, making it cracked and sore. Ask your doctor to examine your baby's mouth as well as your breasts, as thrush may be present there too. There are topical creams that can be prescribed to resolve the infection. During treatment, breast-feeding from the affected side should be stopped temporarily, and expressing carried out instead, either manually or with the aid of an electric or hand pump. Your baby will be able to feed sufficiently from one breast only, as the extra demand will increase the milk supply. Any expressed milk may be given to your baby, or frozen for future use. As the skin heals, breast-feeding can be resumed, but care must be taken that your baby is well positioned and correctly attached on the breast at each feed to minimise any trauma or friction to the nipple. Further assistance with breast-feeding can be obtained from your local breast-feeding counsellor.

**My baby has developed eczema. Could it be something to do with what I ate during pregnancy?**

It sounds as though you are feeling guilty, as if your baby's eczema is your fault. There is no good evidence that what you eat during pregnancy has any effect on the subsequent development of eczema in a baby. Relax – it is not your 'fault'.

## ARE THERE ANY TESTS?

**I have heard a lot about different allergy tests and am confused. My local supermarket offers tests of this kind and a friend has also suggested the ELISA test. Can you give me any more information about these types of test and allergy tests in general?**

'Allergy tests' mean different things to different people and you will hear a lot of conflicting information about their use. Broadly speaking, there are two types of allergy tests applicable to skin disease:

- patch tests;
- skin-prick tests (this type of testing can also be carried out on blood samples with an ELISA test but both of these techniques are testing the same thing).

**Patch tests** look for evidence of contact eczema (also called dermatitis), such as is seen in allergy to nickel, chromate, rubber, dyes, glues or perfumes. This is a delayed allergy that sometimes develops after repeated exposure to a substance. Contact eczema is uncommon in children, perhaps because they haven't had enough exposure to these allergens, so patch tests are not needed (or indeed helpful) in uncomplicated atopic eczema in childhood. Patch tests are complicated to do and interpret (they are done only by specialist dermatologists) but are useful in investigating certain types of eczema – such as isolated hand eczema, especially in people with certain jobs such as hairdressers, builders and nurses.

**Skin-prick tests (or ELISA tests)** look for an immediate type of allergy (Type 1 allergy). There are hundreds of allergens that can be used in these tests but the common ones are pollens (grass and tree), dog fur, cat fur, house dust mite, egg, milk, fish and nuts. They can be useful in detecting relevant allergens in asthma, food intolerance and hayfever. However, they do not provide much, if any, useful information in atopic eczema and most experts in childhood eczema now realise this. The majority of children with eczema have multiple positive results to the skin-prick test, and these are difficult to interpret in any useful way. Children's skin seems hyper-reactive to many substances. Although some doctors still do these tests, we believe that it is unjustified to inflict 15 pin-pricks or a blood test on a young child with atopic eczema if it is not going to provide any practical information in helping to manage the eczema. These tests do not help in deciding whether a certain food might make eczema worse and, if they are wrongly interpreted, can cause problems if nutritional foods are excluded unnecessarily.

**My doctor has refused to do allergy tests on my daughter – can I insist that these be done?**

It sounds as though you and your doctor have a problem.

Words like 'refuse' and 'insist' are very strong, as you need to be able to discuss the investigation and treatment of your daughter's eczema in a calm way. If you read through the answers given above about allergy tests, it might help you to understand why they are not likely to change the way your daughter is treated. This is a very important concept and doctors are often the worst offenders in carrying out tests unnecessarily. With eczema, it is very difficult to justify the pain inflicted on your daughter by having the tests done, and in today's tightly budgeted NHS we have to look at the cost of tests as well as treatment and be able to justify the expense.

## MISCELLANEOUS

**My 3-year-old daughter likes to drink her bath water! Is this dangerous?**

Most toddlers seem to drink the bath water on occasion, and in small quantities this doesn't seem to be harmful, even if you are using a bath oil. Having special toys to play with in the bath, such as a duck or other plastic toys, can distract them from drinking the water. Bath time should be fun for children but obviously there can be a few hazards to avoid. Always use a non-slip bath mat to prevent accidents and, as with any other medications, keep all skin care products out of reach of children – preferably in a high locked cupboard.

**My parents have always recommended massaging mustard oil into the arms and legs of our children to help with strong bone growth. I have a 3-year-old daughter with eczema and am worried that this might make it worse. What should I do?**

We have come across the practice of using mustard oil on the skin in families from Africa and the Indian sub-continent. There isn't any scientific evidence that this practice helps with bone growth but many people are strong believers in it. It is important to try to respect cul-

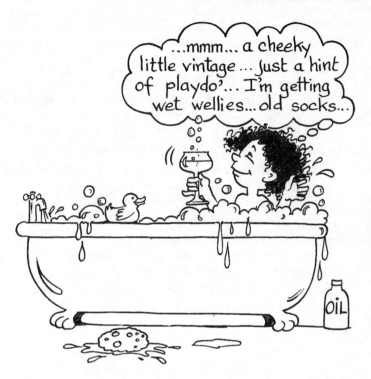

tural practices, as they may be helpful or at least not harmful to eczema. For example, many West Indian and Indian parents use olive oil or aloe vera cream as moisturisers and these seem to be beneficial. Some Nigerian families use hibiscus flower water on the skin; although we are not sure this helps, it certainly doesn't seem to make things worse.

Mustard oil, however, is **very** irritant to the broken skin of eczema and will nearly always make it worse. Because of this, we strongly advise you not to use it. A balanced diet with plenty of calcium and exercise will ensure good bone growth. You will have to explain politely, but firmly, to your parents that mustard oil would make their granddaughter's eczema worse and that she is growing into a healthy girl without it.

**All my children have suffered with bad cradle cap and nappy rash. Why is this and why did they all get better after a few months?**

It sounds as though all your children had seborrhoeic eczema. This is almost universal in babies, in a mild form. It is probably caused by transfer of hormones (androgens) from mother to baby just before birth. These hormones act to stimulate the grease glands (sebaceous glands) of the skin, making them overactive. They are inactive in children until puberty. This hormonal stimulation causes the greasy scaling so typical of this type of eczema. The scalp and nappy area are commonly affected – hence the usual presentation with cradle cap and nappy rash.

As a baby doesn't make these hormones itself and because the transferred hormones are soon broken down and inactivated, the problem of seborrhoeic eczema resolves completely on its own in a few months.

# CHAPTER 3

## Complications of eczema

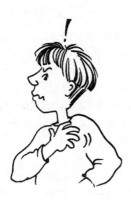

Before moving on to talk about the treatment of eczema, we thought a short chapter on complications would be useful. Most of these relate to infections of one type or another and reflect the fact that eczema causes the skin to lose its barrier function and also that bacteria find it easier to stick to dry, flaky skin. In some cases infection can be serious because not only can 'germs' and irritants pass through the skin but also too much fluid and heat can pass out of the body. In the worst and, thankfully, rare case a child with eczema can quickly become very ill and require admission to hospital.

## BACTERIAL INFECTION

**My GP says that my child's eczema is infected. What causes this and is it dangerous?**

Most cases of infected eczema are due to bacteria. The commonest bacterium to do this is *Staphylococcus* but

33

occasionally another bug called *Streptococcus* causes infection. Bacterial infection may make your child's eczema worse, so it is important to recognise and treat it quickly, but it is not otherwise dangerous as it almost never spreads to other parts of the body.

### How can I tell if my son's eczema is infected?

Infection is a common complication of atopic eczema. If eczema has become very weepy and wet (especially in the joint flexures – e.g. the creases in front of the elbows or behind the knees), if yellowish crusts have formed or if his eczema has suddenly worsened, this may signify infection. If in doubt, you should see your family doctor.

### Is eczema infectious?

No, eczema is an inherited condition that can't be passed on to somebody else. Even when eczema becomes infected with bacteria, this infection does not pass on readily to other people because their skin will be effective in stopping the bacteria getting in.

### My child has eczema of the scalp. Why does he get lumps on the back of the head?

This is almost certainly due to enlargement of the glands (lymph nodes) that are found at the back of the head. These glands are probably swollen due to bacterial infection of the scalp eczema because they act as factories where extra white blood cells are produced to fight the infection. Once the infection is treated the glands slowly shrink back again, but this can sometimes take many months.

We should mention that scalp ringworm (a fungal infection) will also cause these lumps at the back of the head. Scalp ringworm has become very common in children recently and the presence of any discharge from the scalp, whiteheads (pustules) or any hair loss can all suggest this to be the diagnosis. Your doctor can do some tests to check what kind of infection it is, as the treatment of a fungal infection is very different from the treatment of infected eczema.

# ECZEMA HERPETICUM, WARTS AND MOLLUSCUM

**What is eczema herpeticum?**

This is the term that is used for a severe, widespread skin infection with the herpes virus that occurs occasionally in people with eczema. Herpes infections are usually localised, causing a few blisters or a cold sore on the lip. Eczema herpeticum shows much more widespread blistering of the skin and also 'punched-out' sores, which look like little holes in the skin. Typically it involves the face but can occur anywhere on the body. Multiple punched-out, crusted lesions around a patch of eczema should make you suspicious. It is sometimes, but not always, associated with a high temperature and the sufferer may feel quite unwell. Rarely, it can be a very severe infection – especially if the diagnosis is delayed – and it may require hospital admission. Although it is said to have caused death on one or two occasions, we believe that this is very rare, because most parents will seek medical help for their sick child before such a risk arises.

Eczema herpeticum is said to occur because some people with eczema don't fight off the virus very quickly and, furthermore, the scratching and skin damage may help spread the virus. Fortunately, it is a rare complication and easily treated with a medicine called aciclovir, taken by mouth. When problems do arise they are due to failure to recognise the infection, so it is important for you to know what it looks like.

**Are warts more common in children with eczema?**

Early studies suggested that this was the case. However, the results probably reflected a bias in the selection of children for the studies, and current views no longer support this. Viral warts are very common in all children, especially on the hands and feet. They are often noticed in children with eczema because such children are already being seen by doctors about their eczema. However, whilst warts might not be more common, there is some evidence that they are more numerous in children with eczema. This is probably because scratching often aids their spread.

The good news is that warts do not last any longer in children with eczema. They will eventually disappear with no treatment, sometimes after only a number of months.

**My child has had eczema for three years. She recently developed a new rash, which our doctor said was molluscum. What is this?**

Molluscum, also called molluscum contagiosum, are a type of tiny wart in the skin that look rather like small translucent blisters. They are caused by infection with a pox virus. Some people refer to them as 'water warts' although they are in fact solid. They are dome shaped and often have a small depression on the top. Molluscum are very common in all children but tend to be more widespread in those with eczema, probably because the scratching makes them spread. Some of your child's friends may have the same problem.

## GROWTH

**My daughter is smaller than the other girls in her class. Could this be due to her eczema?**

There may be a number of explanations for this. Small stature tends to run in families and this is the most common reason why children are smaller than their friends. Eczema can cause growth suppression but only if it is severe and difficult to control over a long period of time. Other factors to consider with your daughter are whether she has been on a restrictive diet and the medication she has been using. Steroids taken by mouth for longer than a few weeks can certainly suppress growth. Topical steroids are normally without this side-effect unless very strong Group 2 steroid creams (see Chapter 4) are used for many months. Growth delayed by eczema normally catches up when the eczema is controlled.

You must be careful not to just blame eczema as the cause of poor growth. Doctors have height and weight charts for children and your daughter's progress can be charted to see if it is normal. If it is not normal and none of the above situations applies, other rare conditions such as food malabsorption and growth hormone deficiency may have to be considered as possible causes. Your GP might then refer her to a paediatrician.

## OTHER PROBLEMS

**My son has eczema and has developed what looks like a shaving rash on his legs! Can we still apply his creams?**

Yes, but it sounds as though your son has developed a complication of the treatment rather than of the eczema itself. If very greasy, heavy moisturisers are used, they sometimes block the hair follicles and cause folliculitis, which looks like a shaving rash. This is more common if paste bandaging is being used on top of the creams or if the weather is hot and sticky. To avoid this complication, try the following.

- Use lighter moisturisers (see Table 2, in Chapter 4).
- Apply moisturisers by wiping on a thin layer. Don't massage in. Wipe on in the same direction as the hair growth (i.e. **down** the arm and **down** the leg).
- Use steroids in a cream rather than an ointment base.
- Have a break from bandaging until the rash has settled.

If the rash becomes infected, antibiotics may be needed, so watch out for any sudden worsening or general redness. Take him to see his doctor if this happens.

**The teacher complains that my child falls asleep during lessons. Is his eczema to blame?**

If your child's eczema has become out of control, he may be up most of the night scratching and this will certainly make him sleepy the next day. If you are using an antihistamine medicine at night as part of his eczema treatment, the dose may be too high or given too late and either of these could also lead to sleepiness the following day. If the dose is too high, you should be able to adjust it accordingly to make him sleepy just at night-time. If your child is not awake at night scratching or on an antihistamine, you can't blame the eczema!

## IT CAN BE SERIOUS

**My daughter had to be admitted urgently to hospital because her eczema was bad and she became very floppy and ill. I thought eczema was 'just a skin disease'.**

It sounds as though your daughter's eczema has been very severe. Sometimes, if a large area of the body is affected by eczema you can lose too much heat and water from the body. The water loss may be obvious with wet, weepy skin or may be hidden as it just evaporates from hot red skin. Hot skin also loses fluid from the body and children can become ill from dehydration very quickly. The skin is the largest organ in the body and if it 'fails' urgent treatment is needed. Eczema is one of several different diseases that can make the skin hot and red all over. Doctors call this **erythroderma**.

# CHAPTER 4

## Treatment of eczema – 1

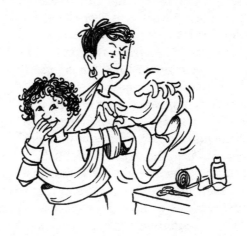

There are many different treatment approaches for eczema, and wherever possible they should be tailored to the individual child and family. It is the parents and the child who actually have to do the treatments. These can be messy and time consuming, and some parents may have to spend two to three hours each and every day applying them, so an appreciation of the hard work involved is important. As a number of different therapies may be equally valid, it is also important that parents are involved in making the decision about which treatment best suits their child. We find that this leads to better motivation and compliance with what can be quite arduous regimens. It is vital that you understand at an early stage that no treatment (conventional or complementary) will **cure** eczema. The ideal aims of treatment are to control the eczema to a level that doesn't interfere in the normal development of a child. This may mean not clearing the eczema altogether, which in the most severe cases can be unrealistic.

A final point to mention is that, however good the treatment is, eczema **will** fluctuate in severity and flare-ups will occur from time to time. This does not mean that the treatment has failed but is just the natural history of the disorder. It is best for parents to have a **two-tier** approach: a more intensive and stronger treatment regimen for flare-ups and a weaker regimen for **maintenance** therapy when the eczema is in a quieter phase.

This first treatment chapter is divided into three sections. '*General Measures*' includes advice on how to avoid environmental factors that may make eczema worse. '*Specific Topical Therapies*' discusses the role of creams and ointments, which are applied direct to the skin, and their role in the treatment of eczema. '*Chronic Eczema – Approaches to Therapy*' deals with some extra therapeutic options that are useful in attempting to break the itch–scratch cycle. This includes behavioural therapy and the role of bandaging. It is a good idea to keep a written record of all the treatments your child has had, so that you can easily show a different GP or consultant what has been tried in the past.

# GENERAL MEASURES

**Since my son developed eczema I have been told not to use soap on his skin. I don't really feel he is clean unless I have used a soap. Can you suggest one that I can use?**

All soaps tend to be irritant to the skin as, by design, they remove not only dirt but also the protective **grease** produced by the skin to maintain its barrier function. We only have to look at the hands of people who do a lot of washing up and cleaning to see how irritant soap can be, so it should be avoided by anyone with eczema. A soap substitute such as aqueous cream is a perfectly adequate cleanser, and you should try using this and see how you get on. If your son or

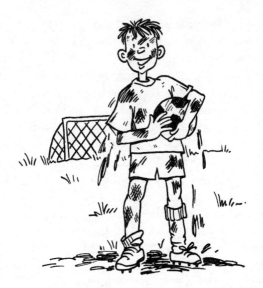

you are set on using a soap, the pH-neutral varieties or the non-perfumed soaps with moisturising creams are preferable to normal soap.

## Can you give me some advice about diet and eczema?

A number of research studies have examined the role of diet in atopic eczema. They have looked at exclusion of dairy products, chicken, wheat, flavourings and additives. Some studies seem to indicate a link but many of the newer studies do not show any relation. You have to remember that all studies in eczema are difficult for three reasons:

- First, eczema fluctuates in severity, regardless of treatment given.
- Secondly, eczema spontaneously resolves in most children as they get older.
- Finally, it is difficult to accurately quantify or score the severity of eczema.

Trials have to take all these factors into account and ideally use a **placebo** group, who receive no active treatment. The placebo group is important because one must know how many people would improve even though they are not getting the specific treatment being assessed in the trial.

This all seems rather confusing but the most recent studies have been well conducted and used placebo groups. They have looked mainly at dairy-free diets and very severe exclusion diets, such as elemental diets in which only a few types of food are allowed. The results have shown that dietary changes do not usually cause an improvement in eczema after the age of one year. There was a possible benefit from a dairy-free diet in children under one year old but the effect was so small that, statistically, this might have occurred by chance. All studies have revealed that it is difficult for families to stick to special diets, especially when children go to school or to parties. We do not therefore routinely advise dietary manipulation as a way of treating eczema.

### Would you ever use a diet?

Yes, we would occasionally consider a dairy-free diet in a child under one year if other conventional treatments were not working well. Also, if there were a clear-cut history of a certain food making eczema worse every time it was consumed, we would consider a three-month exclusion trial.

**Any** dietary approach must be supervised by a dietician to ensure that adequate nutrition is provided. A dietician can also give you invaluable advice on which foods to use and where to get them. Do **not** try to follow diets listed in magazines or shown on television. In our experience, most people who do this develop a regimen that doesn't succeed in completely excluding the relevant food and they are in danger of under-nourishing their child.

We wish that diet was more important in eczema, as it would provide an easy and safe approach to therapy. Our general experience has shown that diets are extremely hard work for parents, and are often disappointing in terms of any impact they have on the eczema.

**My child has eczema and is very allergic to peanuts. Are these two conditions related?**

No, they are probably not directly related. Nuts, especially peanuts, are well known to cause a severe allergic reaction, called anaphylaxis, characterised by swelling of the lips and face, vomiting, difficulty in breathing, a widespread 'nettle rash' and even collapse. The incidence appears to be increasing and the allergy is lifelong, unlike many other childhood food intolerances.

There is a growing feeling that children – especially those with an 'atopic tendency' – should avoid eating peanuts and, to a lesser extent, other nuts until late childhood. This may prevent nut allergy developing but has nothing to do with the causes of eczema.

**Should I remove foods containing colourings and additives from my daughter's diet?**

Unless there is a very strong link that every time these are consumed they make the eczema worse, we do not think this is necessary. Colourings and additives may be important in some children with another skin disorder called **urticaria** or **hives,** but the link with eczema is very tenuous. In practice, they are extremely difficult to avoid, as they seem to be added to so many of the foods favoured by children. You would need to see a dietician for advice before embarking on such an exclusion diet.

**Is there anything else we can do to stop the eczema getting worse?**

Other general measures include:

• Avoiding any pets with furry or hairy coats, such as rabbits, hamsters, dogs, cats and horses.

- Clothes and bedding should be of cotton or even silk, as these are less irritant than wool and synthetic materials (see Appendix 2).
- Keep finger nails cut short and consider the use of cotton gloves or mittens at night.
- Non-biological washing powders may be preferable to biological ones, but the most important factor is that clothes must be rinsed thoroughly after washing to remove traces of these soap powders. An extra rinse cycle on machine washing is useful.
- Pollen can sometimes make eczema worse. Therefore, if you have a garden try to cut the grass in the evening after children have gone to bed.
- When doing housework, vacuuming, polishing or dusting, keep children out of the room where you are cleaning.
- Keep your child cool – hot children sweat and this is irritating, leading to intense itching from dry eczematous skin.
- Don't let your child handle or prepare irritant foods such as citrus fruits, onions, chillies, raw vegetables (especially tomatoes) and salty foods.
- Finally, cigarette smoke can be irritant to eczema so try to persuade smokers to keep their habit outside the home.

## SPECIFIC TOPICAL THERAPIES

A **triple therapy** approach to treating eczema is suitable for most children. This entails:

- a soap substitute and bath oil for washing;
- regular use of a moisturiser;
- intermittent use of the weakest possible topical steroid.

**My mother-in-law says I shouldn't bath my daughter more than once a week because this will make her eczema worse. Is this true?**

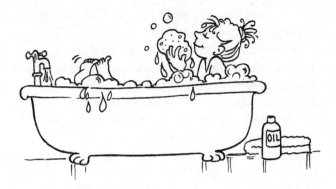

No, we do not agree with this. It is important to wash children with eczema to remove the dry skin scales and the crusts. This helps cut down infection and allows therapy to be absorbed better. Your daughter probably also enjoys having a bath.

However, you **must** add a medicated oil to the bath to prevent the skin drying. Also you should use a non-irritant soap substitute to cleanse the skin, such as aqueous cream or emulsifying ointment. All soaps and any other bath additives such as bubble bath must be avoided because they can irritate the skin. Keep the bath water cool or warm rather than hot, as hot skin tends to dry out more quickly and feel itchy.

### What are pH-neutral soaps and are they better?

Normal soaps have a high pH (see Glossary) because they are alkaline; pH-neutral soaps have a lower pH and are therefore somewhat less irritant. However, soap substitutes such as aqueous cream are better still for people with eczema because the pH of the skin varies from site to site on the body.

### Are there any differences between the bath oils used in eczema?

They are actually very similar, and there is little to choose between them. They are all helpful in allowing the skin to be washed without drying it out. Having said that, some children prefer one to another so there is no harm in trying out the different makes. Some of the bath oils contain tar, which can be soothing, but they don't suit everybody with eczema and some children find the smell unpleasant. Aveeno bath oil contains oatmeal which some children like, but we remember one young boy who described the Aveeno sachet preparation as 'bath sick'!

Some of the newer bath oils have antiseptic properties. These are useful for children with eczema who get recurrent infection of the skin. However, we would not advise all children with eczema to use these continually as there may be a small risk of becoming allergic to one of the antiseptic ingredients.

One of the most useful aspects of using a bath oil is to stop your child putting in a bubble bath, because it contains detergent. Some parents keep the bath oil in an old bottle of the favourite bubble bath, as it is easier than saying 'No'!

**Table 1**   *Bath oils commonly used for eczema*

| MANUFACTURER | NAME |
| --- | --- |
| Stiefel | Oilatum, Oilatum plus,* Polytar Emollient† |
| Quinoderm | Hydromol Emollient |
| Dermal | Emulsiderm,* Psoriderm† |
| Crookes | Bath E45 |
| Merck | Balneum, Balneum Plus, Balneum with Tar |
| Bristol-Myers | Alpha Keri Bath |
| Bioglan | Aveeno (with oatmeal) |
| Schering-Plough | Diprobath |

* has antiseptic properties
† with tar

**What is the difference between a moisturiser and an emollient?**

There is no difference. 'Emollient' sounds somewhat more medical but these words are interchangeable.

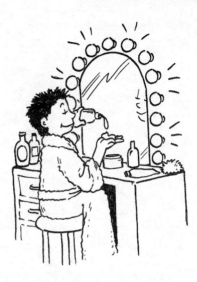

## How much moisturiser should I use on my son?

You should be using as much as is needed to prevent your son's skin from drying out, as that is what makes it more itchy. You or he may need to apply moisturiser five or six times a day if the eczema is severe. We often hear parents complain that their doctor won't prescribe sufficiently large quantities of moisturisers. It would not be unusual to use 500 g or more of a moisturiser in one week or two weeks, depending on the size of your son.

Remember to use the moisturiser to **prevent** the skin from becoming dry. Do **not** let the skin dry out before applying the moisturiser or it will become more itchy. You should be applying it to all the skin – not just the bits with eczema.

## How do I use the moisturiser on my child?

Moisturiser should be applied in a thin layer, wiped on and allowed to soak in. Do **not** rub it in vigorously as this tends to create more itching. A little and often is best. If your child can sit quietly after application the cream will soon soak in.

**Table 2**   *Moisturisers used in eczema*

|  | MANUFACTURER | MOISTURISER NAME |
|---|---|---|
| Very greasy | (generic) | white soft paraffin/liquid paraffin (50:50 WSP:LP) |
|  | (generic) | emulsifying ointment |
|  | (generic) | oily cream (hydrous ointment) |
|  | Schering-Plough | Diprobase ointment* |
|  | Yamanouchi | Dermamist spray |
|  | Bioglan | Epaderm |
| Greasy | Merck | Unguentum Merck cream |
|  | Neutrogena | Neutrogena Dermatological Cream* |
|  | Schering-Plough | Diprobase cream |
|  | Schering | Ultrabase cream |
| Less greasy | Bioglan | Aveeno cream* |
|  | Crookes | E45 cream |
|  | Yamanouchi | Lipobase cream* |
|  | Stiefel | Oilatum cream* |
| Very light | (generic) | aqueous cream |

* not available in 500 g (or equivalent) quantities
('generic' means the chemical or ordinary name of a moisturiser rather than the manufacturer's trade name of its own brand)

## Is it better to use a cream or an ointment?

The easy answer is that an ointment is better unless the skin is very wet and weepy, when a cream is best. Most treatments for eczema are available as creams or ointments and sometimes as lotions. Creams tend to have a high water content and are very easily absorbed into the skin. Once this has happened the skin can often feel just as dry as it did before. Creams therefore need to be applied very frequently – often once or twice an hour. Ointments are much greasier, are not absorbed so well so tend to stay on the surface of the skin and are better at preventing water loss and drying out. They can therefore be applied much less frequently – perhaps as little as once or twice a day. One drawback is that, if the skin is very

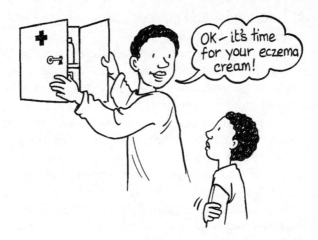

wet, an ointment will simply float on the top and come off very easily.

Unfortunately, real life is not that straightforward and your child may not like the greasier ointments. They do make the skin look greasy, can feel heavy and sticky in hot weather and can stain clothes. It can also be very difficult to use your hands if they are very greasy. The **ideal** moisturiser is probably different for each individual, and the **best** one to use may be the one your child **will** use. The pot of grease that stays on the shelf is useless! Try a variety of preparations with your child – you may find that you end up with a selection, choosing different ones for different parts of the body or times of the day.

### What do steroids do?

Steroids are essentially hormones and there are many different types with quite different actions. The human body makes it own steroids in the adrenal gland and these are vital for the body's normal function.

Different types of synthetic steroids have been developed for use in medicine. There is a group called **anabolic steroids**, which some athletes take (illegally!) to help build up muscle mass, and these should not be confused with the steroids used in eczema.

The other group is called **catabolic steroids** or **gluco-corticoids** (e.g. prednisolone); they are used as an oral medicine for a variety of different diseases because of their anti-inflammatory and immunosuppressive properties. This means that they act by damping down the activity of various immune cells that cause inflammation. Catabolic steroids have proved a very useful medicine, even life-saving, in some medical conditions such as severe asthma or rheumatoid arthritis. The down side of this group of steroids is that if they are used at a high dose **for a pro-longed period** they have many side-effects such as weight gain, bone thinning, decreased growth in children, high blood pressure and loss of muscle mass. Because of this, doctors try to use these at the lowest possible dose for short periods. This type of steroid is occasionally used in the treatment of a very severe flare-up of eczema (see Chapter 5). However, for the reasons already mentioned, they would normally be used for only a few weeks, starting at a high dose and then slowly decreasing. This method should prevent or minimise any serious side-effects.

Fortunately, these anti-inflammatory steroids can also be made into creams for topical application – directly onto the skin. They act in a way like that of their oral counterpart, as they have been developed to try to produce the same anti-inflammatory properties without all the general ('systemic') side-effects on the rest of the body, even after long-term use. This approach has been very successful and the topical steroids provide one of the main components in eczema treatment.

**I'm confused because my neighbour says that steroids will harm my child but the doctor says that hydrocortisone is very safe to use, even on a baby. Why is there so much conflicting infor-mation about steroids and their safety?**

This is an extremely common question and concern of parents. We are not entirely sure why so much mis-information has been generated about topical steroids but people do seem to have extremely strong views about their safety. The anxiety about the use of topical steroids has led to significant under-use of a very valuable form of therapy. This has caused much unnecessary suffering for children. If you talk to doctors who looked after children before the 1950s, when topical steroids were developed, you will realise what an enormous advance they have been in managing eczema.

The following points may in part explain why some of the myths have developed.

- Originally some of the earliest topical steroids developed were very strong, Group 1, steroids (Table 3). These will readily cause skin thinning if used on any skin other than palms and soles. For this reason they are almost never used in eczema. Unfortunately, when this side-effect was first noticed, all topical steroids got a bad name because people then thought mistakenly (and some still do) that the side-effect occurred even with the very weak ones. Remember that topical steroids vary enormously in strength.
- Steroids taken by mouth have many side-effects. Many people assume that topical steroids have them as well. This isn't true. Topical steroids were developed specifi-cally to try to prevent the problems of oral steroids.
- There are different types of steroids: they act differently and have different side-effects. It is easy, though, to assume that all steroids are the same and thus mis-understand the side-effect risks. For example, anabolic steroids can cause an increase in muscle size and liver damage, but this does **not** occur with the topical steroids used in eczema – which are from the glucocorticoid (catabolic) group.

- Many people have become disillusioned with conventional medicine. There has been a social trend to assume that Western medicines are dangerous and that herbal remedies or natural products are safe and preferable. The word 'steroid' has become almost synonymous with all that is bad about conventional medical treatments.
- Steroids do not cure eczema, so it often recurs after using them. You may have expected a cure – partly because the media loves reporting on 'miracle cures' – and might be reluctant to use them again.

## Does this mean that steroids are completely safe?

We would not claim that any conventional therapy is 100% safe but then neither are less conventional treatments. Risks have to be assessed for any form of therapy. If topical steroids are used appropriately, they are an extremely valuable, safe and effective part of eczema therapy. Table 3 gives some of the different types and strengths.

The following list should act as a guideline to the safe use of topical steroids.

- Use steroids only if the eczema is not controlled by moisturisers and bath oils, and use them only for as long as is needed.
- Use steroids only if the eczema is red, itchy and inflamed. Do not use in place of a moisturiser on dry skin.
- Steroids should not be used more than twice daily. Some of the newer steroids are designed for once-daily use.
- In all children, always use weak Group 4 steroids on the face, where the skin is thinner.
- In older children, Group 3 or 4 steroids may be used on the body. Group 2b steroids may be used for flare-ups.
- In older children with very severe eczema, Group 2 steroids are occasionally used on the body. They can thin the skin so they must be used for only a few days.
- Group 1 and 2 steroids are occasionally used for eczema

on the palms and soles, where the skin is very thick. They should not be used on the back of the hands or the top of the feet.

**Table 3** *Topical steroids classified by strength*

| GROUP/STRENGTH | CHEMICAL NAME | TRADE NAME |
| --- | --- | --- |
| 1/Very strong | 0.05% clobetasol propionate | Dermovate |
| | 0.3% diflucortolone valerate | Nerisone forte |
| 2a/Strong | 0.1% betamethasone valerate | Betnovate |
| | 0.025% fluocinolone acetonide | Synalar |
| | 0.1% mometasone furoate | Elocon* |
| | 0.05% fluticasone propionate | Cutivate* |
| 2b/Moderately strong | 0.025% betamethasone valerate | Betnovate RD |
| | 0.00625% fluocinolone acetonide | 1/4 Synalar |
| 3/Moderate | 0.05% clobetasone butyrate | Eumovate |
| | 0.05% aclometasone dipropionate | Modrasone |
| 4/Mild | 0.5% hydrocortisone | (generic) |
| | 1% hydrocortisone | (generic) |

\* once-daily use only

('generic' means the chemical or ordinary name of a steroid rather than the manufacturer's trade name of its own brand)

### My son's skin is lighter in the areas where he has had eczema – is this because of the steroid?

No, it is more likely that the eczema itself has caused a change in pigmentation of the skin. It can either decrease, as in your son, or increase the pigmentation. This problem can occur in anybody with eczema but is much more common in racial groups with pre-existing pigmented skin, such as Asians or African/Caribbeans. This problem is not just confined to eczema. Any inflammatory skin condition (e.g. psoriasis or even acne) can cause pigment disturbance.

If the eczema is controlled, and kept that way, the pig mentation will go back to normal, but this takes a numbe of months.

**People tell me that steroids will thin my daughter's skin. Wha does that mean?**

If very strong topical steroids are used on the skin for mor than a few weeks, they can certainly thin the skin, some times called **skin atrophy**. Topical steroids may be classifie into five groups depending on their strength (see Table 3) The strongest, Groups 1 and 2, are most likely to cause ski thinning. If this happens, the skin looks thin, prematurel aged and may wrinkle. These changes are often reversible i the early stages. With continued application of stron topical steroids, the blood vessels of the skin may becom abnormally widened, or dilated, giving an appearance c stretch marks; this tends to be irreversible. Of cours stretch marks may appear for other reasons, such as th rapid growth of puberty or in pregnancy. The weake topical steroids are used in the treatment of eczema, t avoid thinning especially on the face where it is more likel If stronger steroids are used, it is normally only for a fe days, such as during a flare-up of eczema. Your docto should give you accurate instructions about which steroi to use where, and for how long. Provided these are adhere to, topical steroids can be used quite safely, and skin thir ning is not a significant problem.

**What should I do to prevent the steroid side-effects affecting m child?**

The most important advice here is to stick to the instructior from your doctor about which steroid cream to use wher and for how long. Steroids are the **active** treatment for you child's eczema and should only be needed in the short tern If they aren't working, you should consult your doctor agai and your child may need a different or stronger treatmen

## How do I use a steroid preparation 'sparingly?'

This instruction often causes unnecessary anxiety and, of course, it is far from self-explanatory. All this means is that just enough steroid should be applied to the skin so that a thin glistening layer can be seen after application.

## Can steroids be used on broken skin?

'Do not use on broken skin' is often written on the packaging of topical steroid creams. This is not very helpful and indeed is rather alarmist. It could be said that all children with eczema will have evidence of broken skin by the very nature of the condition. We suspect that pharmaceutical companies are being over-cautious but there is some evidence to suggest that, if very large areas of broken skin are treated, increased absorption of the steroid can occur. However, we feel that topical steroids can still be used safely, provided they are used sparingly (see the previous question), on any patch of eczema even if it is infected – although in that case an antibiotic will be needed as well. Where the skin really is 'broken' (e.g. after a graze), steroids should not be used, because they can slow down healing.

## The eczema around my daughter's eyes is very painful but I am worried about using a steroid in this area. What do you suggest?

If the eczema around her eyes has become painful, this suggests that it is quite severe, uncontrolled and may be infected with bacteria. Infection normally manifests as weeping or crusted skin. There is also a risk of eczema herpeticum (see Chapter 5), as it commonly affects this site. We would advise you to consult your doctor in this situation. If the eczema is infected, you will need treatment with an antibiotic – as either a cream or tablets, depending on the extent of the infection.

Once the infection is being treated, you will also need to treat the eczema. Topical steroids are quite safe in this area provided your daughter keeps to the weaker ones (Group 4). They need to be applied carefully to prevent direct contact with the eyes. The Group 4 steroids will not cause any side-effects; after a few days the eczema should settle down and you may be able to withdraw the steroid. It is unfortunate that most steroids say 'Do not use on the face' on their packaging. This is unnecessarily alarmist.

You should also use a moisturiser regularly around her eyes.

**My teenager is fed up with using steroids to treat her eczema. What are the alternatives?**

If your daughter is fed up with using steroids, she may be using them inappropriately. They are designed for short-term use only, so she may not be using enough preventive treatment (i.e. avoiding soap and using enough moisturiser) or her eczema may need a stronger treatment. Anyone can get fed up with regular treatment and teenagers do tend to rebel against any 'routines' that are imposed on them or affect their developing individuality.

Without knowing the details about your daughter's eczema, it is difficult to discuss alternatives that might be relevant to her. If she just objects to 'steroids' she could try tar preparations but these can be very messy. Some herbal preparations, for example camomile, can help and are discussed further in Chapter 6. Other approaches involve taking tablets or going to hospital, and you should read the sections on these treatments later in the book.

**My son is one of the smallest boys in his class. He has had eczema from early life and has used steroid creams for most of this time. Could they be hindering his growth?**

We would need further information about his condition and treatment to answer this accurately. However, the following factors may be relevant.

If children have severe eczema for many years the eczema

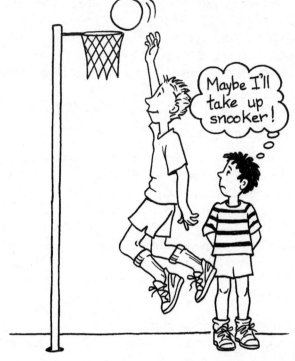

itself interferes with growth. This is true of any chronic inflammatory disorder in childhood. For example, poor growth is also seen with cystic fibrosis or chronic renal failure, in which there is chronic inflammation in the lungs and kidneys respectively. The second possible factor is medication. If your son has had a lot of treatment with **oral** steroids, these will undoubtedly suppress growth. Topical steroids do not usually suppress growth, because little is absorbed beyond the skin. However, if large quantities of strong steroids (Group 2 or 1) are used over a long period or if steroids are used regularly under bandaging or wet wraps, a significant amount may be absorbed and might affect growth. The final factor is the genetic control of growth. Short parents tend to have short children. Also remember that children grow at different rates, especially in early puberty.

When severe eczema does interfere with growth, it is not always permanent. Most of these children will have delayed growth but they usually catch up in later childhood.

# CHRONIC ECZEMA – APPROACHES TO THERAPY

You might find that, despite trying hard to avoid things that make eczema worse and despite employing the **triple therapy** discussed in the previous section, your child still has persistent chronic eczema. The itching, rubbing and scratching have made the skin become dry and thickened – sometimes you may hear it called 'lichenified' – in certain areas. This section discusses some other treatments that can help. They should be regarded as extra treatments to be added to the topical therapies mentioned above.

**My child scratches a lot at night and wakes up every morning with blood on the sheets. He seems much less itchy in the day. Why is this?**

Itching is often worse at night and there could be a number of reasons.

- Children tend to get hot under their bedding, and higher temperatures seem to encourage a feeling of itchiness. You may notice that hot baths also make your child more itchy.
- Another important factor at night is that children are not occupied or distracted by toys or games as they would be during the day. Children seem to concentrate on their skin and get into a non-stop itch–scratch cycle.
- Finally, the presence of house dust mite in bedding and on soft toys (see later this chapter) may be important in making the eczema worse in some children.

## How can I stop my child from scratching at night?

Optimising topical therapies (e.g. topical steroid and moisturisers) should always be the first step. Antihistamine medicine, taken by mouth, can be a useful extra therapy at night as it can help children get off to sleep. Antihistamines come in two types.

- The newer ones, such as Zirtek (cetirizine) and Clarityn (loratadine), which are often used in hayfever, do not cause drowsiness as a side-effect and are of little help in eczema. This is because the itch of eczema is not dependent on histamine.
- The older antihistamines, such as Vallergan (trimeprazine), Phenergan (promethazine), Piriton (chlorpheniramine) and Atarax (hydroxyzine), cause sedation as a side-effect and are more useful in eczema. We are actually using the drug for one of its side-effects rather than its antihistamine properties.

The limitation of this therapy is that it can't be used readily during the day because it makes children too sleepy. The night-time dose must be tailored to the individual child and it may take some days to establish the dose needed. You should give enough to make the child sleepy at night but obviously not so much as to cause the child sleepiness the following morning.

## There are a lot of bedding products on the market at the moment. Can you tell me which is the best one to use?

There are indeed a large number of bedding products. We need to explain about house dust mite (HDM) to understand this approach to treatment. The house dust mite is a microscopic organism invisible to the naked eye and it loves living in soft furnishings. It undoubtedly can make asthma worse but evidence about its role in provoking eczema, although increasing, is as yet limited. It is in fact the house dust mite droppings that cause an allergic response by bringing enzymes from the mite's gut into contact with the skin.

Bedding products are aimed at decreasing the numbers of house dust mite but none will eradicate it altogether. They may be divided into two groups.

- Mattress covers, which stop colonisation by the house dust mite.
- Bedding sprays, which kill house dust mites.

## MATTRESS COVERS

There are a number of mattress covers that are claimed to decrease the numbers of house dust mite in bedding. A recent trial using Gortex mattress, duvet and pillow covers, in combination with regular damp dusting and vacuuming, showed an improvement in some individuals with eczema. (Unfortunately, Gortex is no longer marketed in the UK for mattress covers.) Other trials of bedding covers have been less convincing. They all lead to a decrease in the number of house dust mites but this does not always benefit eczema sufferers.

## BEDDING SPRAYS

There are a number of spray products, called **acaricides**, on the market, aimed at killing mites in bedding. They have a variety of chemical names such as natamycin, benzyl-benzoate, tannic acid, benzyltannate and bioallethrin. They all produce a variable decrease in house dust mite but when used in isolation they rarely have a significant impact on eczema. This may be because they do not get rid of the house dust mite droppings, so repeated washing of bedding is also needed.

Unfortunately, there is no study that has compared the treatment options mentioned above, so we do not know if one is better than another. Also, there are other factors to consider in the house dust mite story. The following tend to increase house dust mite numbers:

- late summer;
- hot, humid conditions;
- older houses;
- older mattresses.

The 'reducing house dust mite' approach requires a lot of effort and has significant cost implications – these products are not available on prescription. The sprays need to be repeated, every 6–12 weeks, and the covers replaced

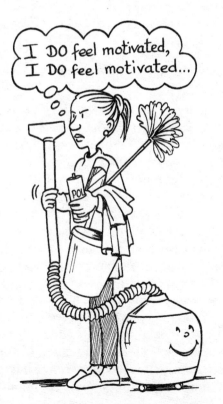

regularly, every 6–12 months. Using one option in isolation tends not to work. A combination of covers, sprays and vacuuming/damp dusting is more likely to be effective but is no guarantee of success. On balance, we feel that, for such a relatively small improvement in eczema, we would not recommend this costly approach as a routine first-line treatment. If eczema is proving to be very severe and unresponsive to treatment and your child also has asthma, it may be worth a trial for two to three months, provided the family is feeling very motivated.

More clinical trial work needs to be done to compare the effectiveness of the different sprays and covers in improving eczema rather than just their ability to remove house dust mite.

A list of manufacturers of bedding products is included in Appendix 2.

### Can you recommend a vacuum cleaner that will get rid of house dust mites?

Most vacuum cleaners help decrease house dust mites (HDM) to some degree from carpets but they will certainly not eradicate them. The modern vacuum cleaners with filters may decrease house dust mite more efficiently but a recent study suggested there is little to choose between the different makes of vacuum cleaner when it comes to improving eczema. In an ideal world it would be better to get rid of carpets and replace them with linoleum, tiled or wood floors. These can then be regularly damp dusted or washed.

However, bear in mind that carpets are not the only good home for house dust mite. All soft furnishings, including sofas, mattresses, duvets etc., harbour house dust mite and it is worth taking soft cuddly toys into account if you are having a real 'blitz'. In fact, bedding harbours more mite than do carpets. Therefore, vacuuming alone is unlikely to have a significant impact on the house dust mite population. Whilst house dust mites may be important in causing asthma, it remains uncertain how important they are in eczema.

**My baby developed eczema at the age of 4 months. She is now 6 months old and on the whole her eczema is under control with topical treatments from the GP. However, her face is always very red and sore, particularly when she wakes up in the morning, despite using moisturisers last thing at night. What should I do?**

It might be worth thinking about the cot and bedding material. Often with a new baby, well-meaning relatives offer you their cots, prams etc., that they no longer require. If this is the case the house dust mite content of a second-hand mattress will be exceptionally high and irritate your baby's face. It would be worth investing in a new mattress if possible and/or a mattress cover.

Always ensure that mittens are worn at night to limit scratching, and that the sheets are soft cotton or silk as it is not uncommon for babies to rub their faces on bedding if they cannot scratch. Other general measures to consider are:

- vacuum the mattress thoroughly at least once a week;
- never use feather pillows or duvets;
- try to use a foam mattress; if this is not possible, use a mattress cover;
- don't put toys or books, or any other item that may collect dust, on shelves above the bed.

**My son seems to have become resistant to the Vallergan I give him at night.**

This does occur quite commonly if an individual anti-histamine is used regularly every night. Children seem to become tolerant to the effect of the drug. This can some-times be prevented by using the Vallergan (trimeprazine) intermittently, keeping it for times when the eczema is flaring up. An alternative strategy would be to change to a different antihistamine such as hydroxyzine (Atarax), promethazine (Phenergan) or chlorpheniramine (Piriton).

Very rarely, antihistamines seem to make children hyperactive rather than sleepy. This doesn't mean that the other antihistamines will do the same, so changing over is the best option.

## BANDAGING

**I have heard that there is some form of bandage used to treat eczema and I wondered if this might be something my 3-year-old daughter would benefit from?**

Paste bandages are sometimes used to treat children with 'difficult' eczema. This may include children with thickened (lichenified) areas of skin on the legs and arms due to chronic scratching. They cannot be used on the trunk. Paste bandages are available on prescription and can be a successful short-term treatment for this problem. One of the advantages of this type of treatment is that they can be applied and left on for up to three days. This reduces the amount of time spent on daily skin care, giving both the parents and the child some respite from the monotony of skin care routines.

Bandaging consists of the following:

- wash your daughter in an oily bath and pat her dry;
- apply her steroid ointment;
- apply an impregnated paste bandage to her limb (see below);
- apply a top bandage, wrapped **around** the limb to hold the lower layer in place.

The impregnated paste bandaging has to be put on in a **backwards and forwards** technique (pleating). It should not just be wrapped around the limb the way a crepe bandage is for, say, a sprained ankle. This technique allows for any drying and shrinkage of the bandage, which might cause constriction of the limb and damage the blood supply. Some skill is needed to do bandaging well but we find that, after one 30-minute lesson with a nurse, many parents become quite adept. With a little practice, most parents can bandage all four limbs within 20–30 minutes.

Bandages should be seen as a short-term treatment of chronic eczema and are often ideal for use a couple of weeks at a time. If your daughter is shy about using them at school, they can be used at weekends or in school holidays. They can also be used just at night if you cannot find the time in the morning for daily application.

### What types of bandaging are there?

There are a number of types of **inner** bandage that are worn directly against the skin. There is little to choose between them, and they can be prescribed by your family doctor. Ichthopaste (zinc paste and ichthammol) and Viscopaste (zinc oxide paste) are the two used most commonly in the UK.

A common **outer** bandage used is called Tubifast. This is a tubular bandage that is available on prescription from GPs and easy to apply. Another type is called Coban but it is not available on NHS prescription. This is a pity because Coban is very useful owing to the fact that it is so difficult to pull off by even the most determined child! Coban can be provided through a hospital pharmacy if your child is under the care of a dermatologist.

### How do bandages work?

Bandages are a useful supplementary treatment for chronic eczema of the limbs. They work in a number of ways.

- First, they provide a barrier to prevent scratching and therefore help to break the itch–scratch cycle.

- Secondly, they provide more of a constant environment for the skin, avoiding changes in temperature and humidity to the skin, which helps lessen itch. (Changes in temperature, such as getting undressed or getting out of a warm bath, often make people feel itchy even if they don't have eczema.)
- Finally, bandaging helps increase the absorption of topical treatments so that they may be more effective.

**What are wet wrap bandages?**

This is a special bandaging technique that can be used to treat all of the skin, including the face. It is usually carried out when children are being treated in hospital. It is difficult, but not impossible, to do at home.

The wet wrap technique involves using two layers of gauze-type bandages, which are cut to fit the limbs, trunk and, occasionally, the face. A steroid cream is applied to the skin or the inner bandage layer. The inner layer is also soaked in warm water, hence the name 'wet wraps', although the top layer is left dry. The bandages have to be changed every 12 hours to prevent drying.

Wet wraps are most commonly used for children who have **erythrodermic** eczema. This is a severe, widespread type of eczema in which more than 90% of the skin is bright red and inflamed. Children may feel quite unwell with a high temperature. Fortunately, it is very rare. The wet wraps are a very useful way of rapidly controlling erythrodermic eczema. A significant amount of the steroid is absorbed so they are normally used for short periods of time – only three to seven days.

There has been a recent trend to use wet wraps with just moisturisers in the treatment of mild eczema. This is probably in response to an inappropriate fear of mild topical steroids. We do not think this is a very realistic approach: wet wrap bandages are not cheap, and the technique can impose a terrific burden on parents. The bandages take a long time to apply and this can increase a child's feeling of being 'abnormal'.

## PSYCHOLOGICAL ASPECTS

**My son scratches constantly even when he doesn't appear to have much eczema. It seems to have become a habit or addiction for him. His eyes glaze over and he keeps scratching until he bleeds. It's almost as though he gains pleasure from this. How can we try to help break this cycle?**

You are not alone! This distressing story is frequently expressed by parents and shows how devastating and disruptive eczema can be for families. The standard eczema therapies should always be optimised as the first step but this may not be effective when scratching has become a habit or a learned behavioural response. Children, and indeed adults, do gain a sensation of pleasure from scratching itchy skin. Chronic under-treatment of eczema can predispose to this situation developing. A lot of research has been conducted recently among dermatologists and psychiatrists at the Chelsea and Westminster Hospital in London on how best to break this cycle.

The first thing to do is to **start again**. Discuss all the options with your local doctor and develop a fresh new approach. Parents should come up with a plan that best suits them and their child, with the aim of taking control of the eczema. **Manage, don't be managed!**

Write a list: irritants, emollients, bathing, topical steroids, infection, antihistamines, bandages. Consider each point in turn and see how it is being handled. Can anything be improved? Consider whether you have a different regimen for flare-ups and for maintenance treatment. Discuss any worries you have about topical steroids.

On top of this a 'behaviour modification' approach can be helpful, even in young children.

- The more time you spend talking and playing with your son and the more he is occupied with activities, the less scratching occurs.
- Encourage your son to clench his fists and count to 30 and to pinch the skin rather than scratch or rub.
- At bed-time or when bathing or applying creams, dress and undress your son quickly and then play with him for 10 minutes. Changes in temperature often induce intense scratching.
- If watching television or videos, try to sit with your son and hold hands.

Time spent with an interested psychologist or doctor can help in modifying behaviour. They often advise using a hand-held counter during the first week, to record how much scratching is occurring. This awareness is helpful in its own right as children and their parents have often become unaware of the size of the problem. If you can find out in which situations your son is scratching and in which he is not, you can try to alter his activities to give him less chance to scratch. It also provides a useful way of monitoring improvement.

Positive reinforcement of a child's good behaviour by his or her parents is also an important part of the process. Negative comments such as 'Stop scratching!' should be

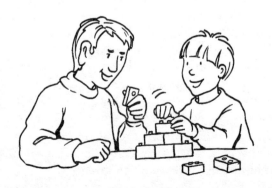

avoided. Positive reinforcement of the whole family from an interested doctor and regular follow-up to monitor progress are also helpful. Set-backs and flare-ups of eczema must be expected. They should be treated promptly and aggressively to continue the improvement in habit reversal.

The behavioural approach can be used successfully in children as young as three years. It is hard work and time consuming for parents and will not suit all families, but the results can be very satisfying. Behavioural therapy should not be seen as an isolated treatment but should be regarded as an extra weapon to be used with other topical therapies in an attempt to break the itch–scratch cycle.

# CHAPTER 5

## *Treatment of eczema – 2*

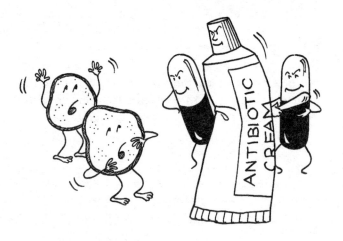

This chapter discusses further treatments and is divided into four sections, dealing with:

- infection;
- treatment in hospital;
- phototherapy (ultraviolet light treatment); and
- treatment taken by mouth.

Whilst infection is a relatively common complication of atopic eczema, the treatments discussed in the other sections of this chapter are relevant to only a small number of children because they are reserved for very severe disease. Of course, severity must be regarded from the child's or parents' perspective and not that of the doctor. The appearance and extent of eczema are not all that should be considered, as the effect it has on a child's life is just as important. Factors such as growth suppression, time off school, severe disruption of sleep and difficulties forming friendships are some of the most important criteria in assessing severity.

# COPING WITH INFECTION

**I think my son's eczema might be infected. Should I still use his steroid cream?**

Yes, you should but the infection also needs to be treated. If infection is very localised, treatment can be with an antibiotic cream or a combination steroid/antibiotic cream. However, infection is often more widespread, so antibiotics by mouth are more appropriate.

Bacterial infection can be caused by either staphylococci or streptococci – two different types of bacteria. The former is much more common, accounting for 90% of cases, and responds well to an antibiotic called flucloxacillin, usually given for 7–10 days. Penicillin is used for streptococci; erythromycin can be used for either if he is allergic to penicillin.

**My daughter has wet eczema. How should this be treated?**

Wet or weepy eczema may be infected so she may well need antibiotic treatment. The wetness is also a sign that the eczema is inflamed, so topical steroids are needed as well but, as discussed in the discussion on 'creams or ointments?' (Chapter 4), a cream formulation should be used.

If her eczema is very weepy on the hands, it can be worth using soaks made up from potassium permanganate crystals or tablets. Standard preparations are available on prescription from your GP. The soaking is done for 20 minutes at a time, twice a day. There are two ways of using the preparations.

- The first is by immersing the hands in the solution.
- The second is by soaking gauze squares or an old flannel

and applying it to the eczema; this allows other areas to be treated as well if they cannot be immersed.

The permanganate solution is antiseptic and also very drying so should be used for **only** two to three days. It tends to stain everything a brown colour – including clothes, sinks and fingernails – so be careful! The fingernails can stay brown for many days but **not** permanently.

**My daughter's eczema keeps getting infected and I am worried about the number of courses of antibiotic she has had. Are there any other treatments we could try?**

Yes, there are some alternatives. One approach is for her to try a topical antibiotic. There are a number of combination steroid/antibiotic creams, which come with different strength steroids. Weak (Group 4) steroid combinations include Vioform-Hydrocortisone (clioquinol and hydro-cortisone) and Fucidin H (fusidic acid and hydrocortisone) cream. These are suitable for use anywhere. Betnovate-C (betamethasone and neomycin), Locoid C (chloroquinol and hydrocortisone) and Fucibet (fusidic acid and beta-methasone) are strong (Group 2) steroids and should only be used for short periods (one to two weeks) in children. They should **not** be used on the face or on children less than one year old.

Whilst the above can help, even topical antibiotics can cause bacterial resistance to develop. Therefore, another approach is to consider the use of antiseptics. These come in bath oil preparations, such as Oilatum Plus (liquid paraffin, benzalkonium and triclosan) or Emulsiderm (liquid paraf-fin, isopropyl and benzalkonium), or as a moisturiser, Dermol 500 (liquid paraffin, benzalkonium, chlorhexidine and isopropyl), and your daughter should be using one of these antiseptic preparations as a preventive measure – see the section on bath oils in Chapter 4. Antiseptic soaps are probably best avoided, as they can irritate eczema. Your daughter should also have swabs taken from inside her nose in case she is harbouring the bacteria there. If so, it can be treated with mupirocin – an antibiotic in a special cream form for use inside the nose.

**My daughter developed eczema herpeticum last year and was successfully treated for it. She is due to start school next month and I know that it is likely that she will come into contact with children with cold sores. Is it possible for her to become infected with eczema herpeticum again? If so, can I do anything to reduce the risks?**

Eczema herpeticum is a rare but serious complication of eczema. Fortunately, it usually occurs only once, but a small proportion of children do suffer with recurrent attacks. However, each episode can be treated the same way with a five-day course of antiviral tablets or liquid taken by mouth.

In general, cold sores are more common in adults than in children but there is still likely to be some exposure at school. In practice it is difficult to prevent exposure to the herpes virus completely because it is so widespread in the community and even at home. If somebody does have an active cold sore, either at home or at school, it is best for your daughter to try to avoid too much close contact, as the virus spreads only by touching. Doting aunts and grand-parents should avoid kissing her if they have an active cold sore, but you will have to explain this to them delicately. School is more difficult, as refusing to sit next to someone with a cold sore may be met by the retaliation of not wanting to sit next to somebody with eczema! This will need to be tackled diplomatically with the teacher to prevent any hurt feelings in the classroom. Once again, it's worth explaining that as long as eczema herpeticum is quickly recognised and treated it is not dangerous.

**How do you treat molluscum contagiosum?**

Molluscum will resolve spontaneously with no treatment

but this takes up to 12 months on average. They can be treated by freezing them with liquid nitrogen but this is very painful and rarely justified, so they are usually left untreated. We would also avoid using liquid nitrogen on Asian or African/Caribbean children as this treatment can permanently alter skin pigmentation.

Old-fashioned treatments include squeezing the lesions with forceps or pricking in some phenol with a needle. We feel that both these methods are painful and can, rarely, cause scarring and so would not recommend them. In most cases the best policy is to leave well alone, so it is only if they are visible and causing distress that we would consider treatment.

## TREATMENT IN HOSPITAL

**My son has bad eczema and has been admitted to hospital twice for treatment. He gets better quickly despite using therapy similar to the one I use at home. Why is this?**

The treatment you use at home probably consists of moisturisers, bath oils and topical steroid creams. Whilst your hospital may have used similar therapy, there are

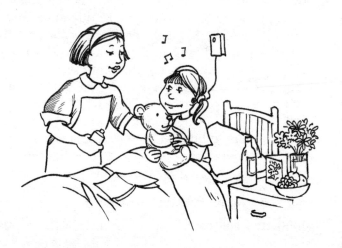

many other differences between hospital and home environments. Eczema is a 'multifactorial' condition – many different factors may be involved in triggering it, keeping it going and making it worse. There may be several reasons why he responds differently in hospital.

- Children often benefit from a change of environment and a fresh approach to their skin, which can have important psychological benefits.
- Children may feel more relaxed, especially if families have developed high levels of stress from disrupted sleep patterns and constant scratching. Playing with the nurses and other children on the ward may provide regular distraction from scratching. Parents may also feel relieved and more relaxed after a break from routine monotonous skin care regimens. Children are very sensitive to parental anxiety.
- Compliance with treatment is usually very high during in-patient treatment even if children are usually rather reluctant and unco-operative.
- Hospital wards have very little in the way of soft furnishings and therefore have less house dust mite than is usually found at home.

In-patient therapy is a useful option when eczema has become very severe. It does not mean that anybody has failed. It provides an opportunity to improve the eczema rapidly, to develop a fresh approach and to give both the child and the parents a well-earned break from the monotony and hard work.

# PHOTOTHERAPY (ULTRAVIOLET LIGHT TREATMENT)

**I have heard that sunshine helps eczema. Will using a sunbed help my child?**

To answer this we first need to explain about ultraviolet light and sunshine. Natural sunlight consists of two ultraviolet wavelengths, called UVA and UVB.

UVB may help to improve inflammatory skin conditions such as eczema. Artificial UVB is occasionally used to treat eczema but only if the eczema is severe and not responding well to standard first-line therapy (see Chapter 4). UVB treatment is carried out only in hospital dermatology departments where doses are strictly controlled. It is given three times a week for a 6- to 10-week course. Sunglasses must be worn during treatment to protect the eyes.

UVA therapy alone is not very effective at treating skin disorders. When it is used to treat eczema, it has to be given with a photosensitising medicine, called psoralen, to make the UVA work more effectively. This psoralen can be given by mouth or applied to the skin in bath water. This treatment is called PUVA therapy, psoralen + UVA. It is given only twice a week but the sunglasses must be worn during the whole of the day of the treatment because the psoralen will continue to sensitise the eyes even to natural sunshine.

Both UVB and PUVA treatment can irritate eczema at the start of treatment. Therefore, to begin with, they are given at very low doses, occasionally with oral steroid 'cover'. The dose is then slowly built up during the course of the treatment. Because these are specialist treatments, they must be carefully monitored.

To return to your question about sunbed usage, most sunbeds are aimed at tanning the skin and consist of predominantly UVA light – so they are not very effective in treating eczema. Moreover, because doses are not measured adequately, more harm than good can be done.

Both UVB and PUVA can cause skin damage, and even skin cancer, later in life if **too much** is given. PUVA carries a higher risk than UVB, so is rarely used in children. For safety, there is a maximum number of PUVA treatments allowed over a lifetime (about 10 courses). These risks of skin damage are much lower for children with Asian or African/Caribbean skin types. Children with pale skin, blue eyes, red hair and freckles are most at risk, so we would not usually recommend phototherapy in this group.

Phototherapy is certainly useful for severe eczema but can be inconvenient, even though the treatment takes only a few minutes each time, because it entails several visits to a hospital department. However, most departments have early morning or late evening appointments, so it shouldn't be necessary to miss school. If this is not convenient for parents, the treatment can be given during the school holidays.

# TREATMENT TAKEN BY MOUTH

This section covers evening primrose oil, systemic steroids, cyclosporin and azathioprine. ('Systemic' drugs are ones that may affect the whole body. They will therefore have an effect on more than the skin. Systemic drugs can be taken by mouth, by injection or by suppository.) With the exception of evening primrose oil, all these therapies are very strong and carry a number of potentially serious side-effects. Their use is restricted to extremely severe eczema that is causing devastating effects on a child's normal development. They should be prescribed (and monitored) only by doctors with expertise in these drugs, and parents must be involved in any decisions about their possible use. Parents **must** understand the potential risks and benefits and the need for monitoring treatment before deciding whether the drugs are appropriate for their child. However, these drugs can dramatically improve children's lives when the eczema has become persistently uncontrolled.

**Will taking evening primrose oil help my son's eczema?**

There are different types of evening primrose oil, made by various companies. To our knowledge the only one that has been used in eczema studies is Epogam. This answer applies **only** to Epogam and may not be applicable to other evening primrose oil preparations, which can have different amounts of the active ingredient in them. The active ingredient is gamma-linoleic acid, of which 40 mg is present in adult capsules and 80 mg in paediatric capsules. Many different makes of evening primrose oil are listed as having 500 mg of oil in them – this is the oil and not the amount of active ingredient. Some studies suggest that 20–30% of people with eczema may gain some benefit with Epogam. It must be given at high dose (4–6 adult capsules per day or 2 paediatric capsules per day) for three months to know if it will work. Other studies have not shown any benefit. Our personal experience suggests that this treatment works best in children with a predominant pattern of dry, flaky skin rather than red, inflamed skin. If your son has that pattern, it may be worth a trial but generally the response is disappointing. It is certainly a very safe treatment. It is interesting to note that breast milk contains much higher levels of gamma-linoleic acid, the active ingredient of evening primrose oil, than is present in formula feeds or normal food.

**The dermatologist has suggested that cyclosporin may help in my child's eczema. Can you tell me some more about this?**

Cyclosporin is a new drug for severe eczema. It is a strong drug with potentially serious side-effects, so you must be sure about the risks and benefits.

It acts by suppressing a chemical called interleukin-2 (IL-2), which is a part of the body's immune system. Because it doesn't affect all of the immune system in the way that steroids given by mouth do, the risks of infection while on this treatment are lower. There doesn't seem to be any increase in bacterial infections while on treatment, but there may be a small risk of the child getting some viral infection such as herpes. The risk, however, certainly seems to be low.

The two main serious side-effects that can occur are high blood pressure and kidney damage. Both of these seem to be reversible when the dose is decreased or the therapy is stopped, so, provided your child is monitored closely, cyclosporin can be used relatively safely. The problems with kidney damage seem to be more common in older people who have been taking the treatment for longer than six months. There are a number of other lesser side-effects, including pins and needles in the fingers, a mild tremor and nausea. However, these seem to improve despite continuing therapy. The final side-effect is an increase in hair growth and an enlargement of the gums. The latter tends to occur in people with poor dental hygiene, so regular dental check-ups are necessary.

Cyclosporin can certainly help severe eczema. The clinical trials suggest that over two-thirds of people taking it can expect an improvement. Our experience is that one-third do extremely well with this treatment – judged by the extent that it can change children's lives. Others get less benefit. We have also noticed that perhaps 15–20% of children have a negligible response. Cyclosporin is still a relatively new therapy for childhood eczema. More research will improve our understanding on the best way to use this drug. It will also bring to light any long-term side-effects that might need to be taken into consideration.

**My friend is taking cyclosporin after a kidney transplant. Why on earth is this used in eczema?**

Cyclosporin is used in transplant medicine to help prevent rejection of the transplanted organ. It acts by damping down the immune system in a rather more selective way than steroids do. Historically, somebody noticed that kidney transplant patients who also had a skin condition called psoriasis found that their psoriasis got much better when started on cyclosporin. It became an approved therapy for psoriasis and was then tried for other inflammatory skin disorders such as eczema. The original studies looked at adults with eczema but now children have also been studied and cyclosporin has been shown to help some of them.

**My son is currently taking cyclosporin for very bad eczema. Will it interact with his other eczema medications?**

Yes, it can. Cyclosporin interacts with a number of oral medicines but not with topical therapies. (By 'interact' we mean that the actions of other medicines can make the side-effects of cyclosporin more likely, or even stop it from working.) Always tell the doctor or pharmacist your son is taking cyclosporin and ask them to check for interactions if any new medicine is being planned, **even** if this is an over-the-counter-preparation. Avoid buying drugs in super-markets where there is nobody to advise you.

- Erythromycin, a commonly used antibiotic, should be avoided **but** penicillin is safe.
- Antihistamines are generally safe.
- Aspirin-type pain killers, used by children over 12, such as Advil, Brufen and Nurofen (which contain ibuprofen) and Ponstan (mefenamic acid) and aspirin itself should be avoided **but** paracetamol is acceptable.
- Finally, if travelling abroad, the antimalarial drug chloroquine can interact with cyclosporin and should **not** be taken.

**My daughter's dermatologist has suggested a course of oral steroids to treat her eczema. How long will she need to take them, and will they cause any side-effects?**

A short course of oral steroids is often used when the eczema has got out of control, as a means of improving things quickly. Most dermatologists use them for a two- to four-week course, often starting at a high dose and then slowly decreasing the dose every few days. Most children do not notice any side-effects when steroids are used this way.

Occasionally, indigestion or weight gain are reported but these should settle down as the steroids are reduced and stopped. Changes in mood – 'depression or euphoria' – can also occur, especially if there was any pre-existing psychological problem, but again this should settle quickly as the steroids are withdrawn.

**My child's asthma was so bad recently that the doctor treated him with steroid tablets. This led to a dramatic improvement in his asthma and eczema. Since stopping them, though, his eczema is getting bad again. Why can't he stay on this treatment?**

Systemic steroids, rather than topical steroids, will usually cause a great improvement, or decrease, of eczema. There are a number of different ways of giving them but you cannot avoid side-effects if they are taken over a long period of time. For this reason they are usually given as a short course to try to control acute flare-ups, both for eczema and for asthma. Eczema will nearly always 'rebound' (worsen rapidly) if systemic steroids are withdrawn abruptly rather than tailing them off; courses for asthma are often given as a high dose for a few days to a week without a reduction before stopping. Other treatments must be put into place to prevent this rebound. These may include topical therapies, antibiotics, phototherapy and so forth.

The side-effects of long-term systemic steroids are many and include:

- weight gain,
- bone thinning,
- high blood pressure,
- diabetes,
- mood changes,
- thinning of the skin,
- growth suppression.

The last side-effect is a particular problem in children, as severe eczema also can cause growth suppression. The most common steroid used is called prednisolone. Occasionally other steroid preparations, such as beclomethasone and budesonide, are used. They cause fewer problems with weight gain and high blood pressure than prednisolone but can still suppress growth. Another medicine, called tetracosactrin (Synacthen), can be used but this has to be given by injection. It is a hormone that makes the body's adrenal glands produce more of its own steroid but has side-effects similar to those of prednisolone. It is usually given as a one-off treatment boost in eczema that is difficult to control.

All long-term steroid therapy comes at a price, and hopefully your son's eczema is not severe enough to make this a price worth paying. It is particularly important to avoid this long-term therapy during puberty, when so much growth occurs. Our own view is that, whilst short-term courses of systemic steroids are useful, long-term use should be the last line of therapy when all else has failed.

## SAFETY FACTORS WITH ORAL STEROIDS

- All children taking oral steroids **must** carry a steroid card or bracelet, giving details of the treatment; it is important for all medical personnel to have this information. The card or bracelet are available from your pharmacist.

- Children taking oral steroids should wait until they are off the treatment before being given 'live' vaccines such as MMR (measles, mumps and rubella), polio (the liquid given with the triple vaccine diphtheria, tetanus and pertussis (whooping cough)) and yellow fever (a travel vaccination).

- Oral steroids should not be stopped suddenly if they have been used for more than four to six weeks. Your doctor will give you a regimen for stopping them gradually. Do not miss doses.

- If there is unrelated severe illness, surgery or trauma, steroid doses may need to be doubled for a while; your doctor will advise you.

- Chickenpox can cause a widespread severe infection in children taking oral steroids. If your child has not had chickenpox and is on oral steroids, avoid contact with known cases of chickenpox or shingles. If such contact occurs, consult your doctor **immediately** for anti-chickenpox immunoglobulin therapy.

### What is azathioprine?

Azathioprine is another very powerful medicine that suppresses the immune system. It works by damping down the bone marrow (which produces blood cells). It can also suppress parts of the bone marrow that have nothing to do with the immune system, so it can cause anaemia or blood-clotting problems. It is used in many branches of medicine as an immunosuppressant for people with kidney transplants, arthritis, inflammatory bowel disease and various skin diseases. Its use in eczema has not been well studied but most dermatologists are convinced that it works; it is used quite commonly in adults with severe disease. It is only very rarely used in children with eczema because of the side-effects. The main worry is bone marrow suppression and liver damage, so anyone taking this drug needs regular blood tests to monitor them. Over all, it probably has fewer side-effects than oral steroids but it remains a last-resort drug for children with devastating eczema.

### Are the tablets used for our daughter's eczema dangerous in overdose?

Yes – it is best to consider all tablets as dangerous in

overdose for children. If she is taking tablets that need careful monitoring, they can be very dangerous indeed. Keep **all** tablets well out of reach and preferably in a lockable cabinet.

# CHAPTER 6

## Complementary therapies

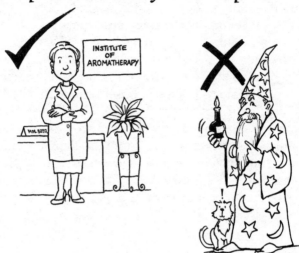

Almost no modern medical book for patients or their carers would be complete without a section on complementary or 'non-conventional' treatments. It is, however, the most difficult area in which to give definite answers to questions. Those who get better with complementary treatments are very positive about it and this can, unfortunately, raise the hopes of parents whose children might not gain the same benefit. You will rarely hear people talking negatively about complementary treatment but we do see people who either don't get better or, sadly, are made worse. Most of the success stories are what we call **anecdotal** evidence, because a proper scientific study has not been carried out.

## CHOOSING A SAFE PRACTITIONER

Most complementary practitioners work privately and are better than NHS doctors at 'selling' their treatment. They also tend to spend more time with patients and there is undoubted benefit in being able to talk about your child's illness and its impact on you. It can be very relaxing to talk – would that we all had more time to spend allowing patients to talk. This is not to say that the only benefit from complementary medicine derives from spending money to buy 'protected time'. Some people do seem to get better and this also applies to children who may gain less psychological benefit than you, their parents. It is worth remembering that 'complementary' is a much better term than 'alternative' as it should sit beside the standard first-line treatments for eczema, not replace them. There are now professional bodies that regulate most forms of complementary treatment and you should contact them before choosing a practitioner. Remember that you don't have to have any medical qualifications to work in complementary medicine, so discuss your plans with your GP so that at least you can check if the complementary practitioner gets the diagnosis right.

### How do I choose a safe complementary practitioner?

The Royal College of Nursing has put together some very sensible guidelines for you to use when thinking about complementary medicine. You should always ask the practitioner:

- What are his/her qualifications and how long was the training?
- Is he/she a member of a recognised, registered body with a code of practice?
- Can he/she give you the address and telephone number of this body so you can check?
- Is the therapy available on the NHS?
- Can your GP delegate care to the practitioner?
- Does he/she keep your GP informed?

- Is this the most suitable complementary medicine for your child?
- Are the records confidential?
- What is the cost of the treatment?
- How many treatments will your child need?
- What insurance cover does the practitioner have in case things go wrong?

Then ask yourself the following questions.

- Did the practitioner answer your questions clearly and to your satisfaction?
- Did the practitioner give you information to look through at your leisure?
- Did the practitioner conduct him/herself in a professional manner?
- Did the practitioner make excessive claims about the treatment?

You should **avoid** any practitioner who:

- claims to be able to completely cure eczema;
- advises you to stop your child's conventional treatment **without** consulting your GP;
- makes you, or your child, feel uncomfortable; you need a good relationship if you and your child are going to get full benefit from the treatment.

## AROMATHERAPY

**I would like to take my daughter to my aromatherapist for a massage as I find it very relaxing and I thought that it might help her cope with her difficult eczema. Would this be a good idea?**

It depends on how bad your daughter's eczema is. Aromatherapy involves the use of essential oils which are aromatic (scented) oils extracted from the roots, flowers or leaves of plants. These oils can cause problems if massaged into the skin, which is the usual way of using them. The massage itself, however, can be very relaxing so, if your daughter doesn't have widespread eczema, it could be worth discussing with the aromatherapist. We would recommend that any oil used is tested on your daughter first by applying a little to her forearm for a few days to rule out any chance of sensitivity. Make sure your daughter wants to try aromatherapy; she may feel uneasy about taking her clothes off if she is sensitive about her eczema.

# REFLEXOLOGY

**What is reflexology and can it be used on children?**

Reflexology is a massage therapy that uses acupuncture points on the feet that represent different parts of the body. The feet are massaged using talcum powder so, unless the eczema is on the feet, it is generally safe for children with eczema. As it involves just the feet, your child wouldn't have to undress so should feel comfortable with the treatment. One problem with eczema is that other people don't like touching the skin, so children really enjoy the touching and contact involved in reflexology. Most reflexologists should be happy to teach you how to do the massage.

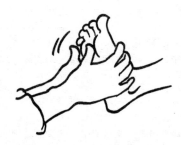

# CHINESE HERBS

**My neighbour says that Chinese herbal medicine has cured her niece of eczema. My 3-year-old daughter has quite mild eczema but it never seems to go away. We would like to try a Chinese herbal treatment but are not quite sure how to go about it – can you help us?**

Chinese herbal treatment comes in two broad categories: creams and oral preparations. The latter is the most commonly used in eczema and has been subject to some preliminary trial work by UK doctors. The following points have come out of these trials.

- There is **no** good evidence that Chinese herbs cure eczema, but they may help improve it.
- Chinese herbs are not always safe and can have short-term side-effects such as causing inflammation of the liver (hepatitis). The long-term side-effects are not known.
- The raw ingredients or herbs are not under any form of quality control. Therefore, the chemical composition may vary enormously, depending on which country the herbs come from, how long they have been kept and, indeed, which time of year they were picked.
- There is a similar lack of control over the 'doctors' who sell them. Chinese herbalists are not medically qualified Western doctors under the control of the General Medical Council. Whilst many Chinese herbalists are responsible people, anyone can sell these herbs. A lot of money can be made by herbalists, bearing in mind the treatment costs £20–£30 per week per patient.
- Preparation of the herbs can take up to two hours, twice a day. The resulting black liquid has to be drunk, but unfortunately tastes quite disgusting. Many children, especially those under five years old, often refuse to take this therapy.

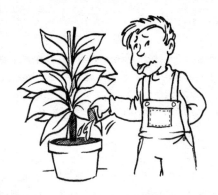

In conclusion, we never recommend this treatment to individuals with mild or moderate eczema, because of the possible toxicity. Herbal treatment may be considered but only when eczema continues to be very severe despite optimum therapies, especially if other potentially toxic (conventional) therapies, such as oral prednisolone or cyclosporin, are also being considered.

It is important that everyone concerned is aware of the risks and of the need for monitoring, by regular blood tests, before embarking on herbal treatment. The expense should also be borne in mind by parents, as treatment with Chinese herbs will often be for six months or longer. Stopping Chinese herbs early often leads to a severe flare-up in eczema, akin to suddenly stopping steroid therapy.

Undoubtedly, Chinese herbs can help eczema in some individuals, and our hope for the future is that the active ingredient(s) will be isolated and developed into less toxic regimens. Finally, remember that your daughter is very likely to grow out of her eczema as she gets older.

## OTHER HERBAL TREATMENT

**Are there any non-Chinese herbal remedies?**

Yes, there is a strong tradition of Western herbal medicine, its roots going back into folklore. There seems to be less published work on this form of herbal treatment and very little scientific evidence that can be accepted by those with a **conventional** approach to treatment. Once again, however, most herbalists will spend time taking a careful history and use creams that are soothing and act as a good emollient if nothing else.

Many of our modern medicines are, in fact, derived from the study of traditional plant-based remedies but an active ingredient has to be identified and thoroughly tested to ensure its safety before it can be licensed as a drug. This may ignore the beneficial effects of a group of extracts working together. You must remember, however, that the skin of many people with eczema is very irritated by contact with plants and side-effects are possible. Check that any herbalist you visit is backed by a professional body and test any new cream on a small area of your child's skin. One herbal preparation that has been studied more than most – and compared to hydrocortisone in some trials – is camomile. There does seem to be some evidence that it has a specific action in improving eczema in addition to a simple moist-urising effect. Tea-tree oil is also growing in popularity and has useful antiseptic properties, but has not been well studied in eczema.

# HOMOEOPATHY

**My friend sees a homoeopathic doctor instead of an ordinary GP. What is homoeopathy and would it help my son's eczema?**

Homoeopaths believe that the symptoms of a disease are actually the body's way of fighting the illness. Rather than trying to reduce the symptoms, homoeopathy tries to work with the body and add to its own healing powers. The 'remedy' prescribed is a minute dose of a substance that, in a normal dose, would produce the same symptoms in a healthy person. The remedy is produced by diluting the substance many times so that no more than a trace is present and the resulting treatment is safe and usually free of side-effects. It is very difficult to say whether your son would benefit from a homoeopathic approach, as there are no good scientific studies showing benefit in children. In our experience we have found it disappointing but he is unlikely to come to any harm.

**Is seeing a homoeopath very expensive?**

Homoeopathy is one of the complementary treatments you can have on the NHS: there are five homoeopathic hospitals in Britain – Bristol, Glasgow, Liverpool, London and Tunbridge Wells. It is between you and your GP whether you can be referred but, if it cannot be arranged, or you feel it would be too far to travel, you can see a practitioner privately; charges might start from around £20 or £30. You do not need a prescription for homoeopathic remedies; they can be bought from a pharmacy and some pharmacists have qualifications in basic homoeopathy. You can get more information from the Homoeopathic Society (see Appendix 2).

# HYPNOTHERAPY

**My son seems to be addicted to scratching; could hypnotherapy work for him as it stopped me smoking?**

This is a very sensible question and we are sure many parents will agree that scratching can seem to be a habit. There have been some studies of hypnotherapy and eczema that have shown some benefit in decreasing the need to scratch, though little objective benefit was seen when the skin was examined in the short term. We don't think it unreasonable to suggest that, if individuals feel better, their skin will benefit from less scratching in the long term. Some GPs have an interest in hypnosis and it is relatively easy to learn a simple form of self-hypnosis. This can make visualising the urge to itch as being controlled by a 'thermostat',

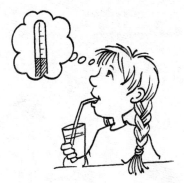

which can be mentally turned down to reduce the itch, as you would turn down a real thermostat to reduce the temperature. Children over 10 can respond well to hypnotherapy, and a modified form involving story telling can be used in younger children. This uses their imagination and susceptibility to suggestion by getting them involved in a story dealing with eczema and allowing them to feel positively about the condition.

## CONCLUSION

In summary, many people benefit from a complementary approach to treatment. Whether this is because of a **whole-person approach** or a really effective therapy is still open to debate. However, if your child gets better without any adverse effects, does it matter? We think that it **does** matter, because the only way these different approaches can become available to all is through acceptance into the NHS and, for that, much more scientific evidence is needed. Whether the necessary research will take place is doubtful; it is very expensive and money can only be made from a patentable new drug not from a natural remedy.

# CHAPTER 7

## Feelings, family and friends

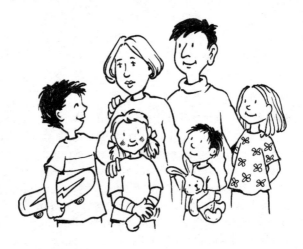

'This is the great error of our day, that physicians separate the soul from our body, the cure of the part cannot be attempted without treatment of the whole.'

This statement reflects many of the criticisms we hear about approaches to treating eczema, and it is particularly true when dealing with children. The 'whole' can be expanded to include the family who, all too often, can feel as if their life is centred on one child with eczema. The surprising thing about the quotation is that it is from Plato in 320 BC and the criticism is just as deserved today as it seems to have been in his day. As we have said earlier in this book, it is impossible to determine the severity of eczema without taking into account its effect on a child's life. You cannot afford to look at the skin in isolation. A recent study reported in the *British Journal of Dermatology* found that children with atopic eczema had twice the rate of psychological disturbance as those with only minor skin problems such as warts.

# FAMILY CONFLICT

**Since my daughter developed eczema, my whole life has revolved around her. Does this happen to other families? What can I do?**

Indeed it does, and knowing that you are not alone is often a help. You could consider making contact with other families to share your feelings and worries. The National Eczema Society can be a useful source of contacts.

Children can be very manipulative, even without an illness to work with. Think of your response when your daughter is scratching. Will you stop doing everything else to deal with her? If you do, what message could this give to her and to other members of your family? It is these sorts of issues that can need the skills of a psychologist or family therapist to deal with. If you find you need help, start by talking to your GP on your own, without your daughter.

**I have a child with bad eczema and this has come to dominate my life. Nobody seems to understand the problems I have to**

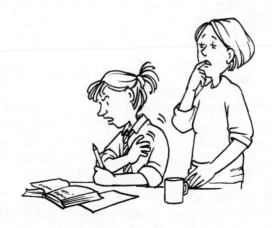

**deal with and the lack of sleep. Is there anyone I could talk to about living with eczema?**

Yes, initially you could talk to your doctor or specialist about the problems with your child's eczema. In the longer term we recommend that you join the National Eczema Society (NES), which has fully trained information staff and 180 'Contacts' around the UK. 'Contacts' are people who have been through experiences similar to yours and will provide you with support over these problems. It is difficult for people to understand how bad eczema can become unless they have some personal experience of it. This is why the NES Contacts have proven to be so useful. You can also meet other sufferers who are not acting as Contacts but with whom you can swap stories and ways of coping. You soon find out that you are not the only one with the problem, which is a help in itself.

**My husband refuses to help with our son's eczema treatment. How can I get him more involved?**

Most of the burden of caring for children seems to fall on mothers in our society, and you may have been to the doctor with your son much more than your husband and so understand much more about the eczema. It is difficult to be specific in your case but here are a few thoughts.

- Is your husband confident about treating your son's eczema? He may be concerned about 'getting it wrong'.
- Does he resent the amount of time you spend with your son at his expense?
- Does the eczema seem to come from one side of the family? If it is from his, he may feel guilty, or if from yours, he may feel it is your problem.
- If you have other children, does he feel he should ensure that they also have quality time with a parent?

We can't give you any simple answers, as you need to discuss the problem in much more detail with your husband and your family doctor or perhaps a dermatology nurse. If your son is old enough, get him to ask Dad to help. It might work.

# MAKING FRIENDS

**My son doesn't seem to make friends easily. How can I help?**

Some children don't make friends easily, regardless of any health problems, so his eczema may be a side issue here. All children are different and it is important not to put pressure on children to match up with what you may see as a 'normal' number of friends. One or two close friendships may be important for one child whereas another might need a large social circle. Talk to your son and find out what his needs are. You can also encourage him to talk about any problems with friendship and gently explore his feelings about teasing, bullying or being 'different' that may be a problem. If he is at school, talk to his teacher who may have some helpful suggestions. The National Eczema Society is a useful source of help, as you can meet other families with children the same age and compare thoughts and experiences.

**My son's eczema is so bad that he refuses to leave the house – can you help?**

All eczema sufferers will find it difficult to cope at times. Children can often find it extremely hard to cope emotionally, especially if they are being teased or bullied at school. Talk to his teacher to find out if there have been any particular incidents that might have upset him, and talk to your son to find out what is bothering him. Eczema can cause misery for the sufferer as well as adding stress to other family members. It is very useful to enlist the help of your 'primary health care team'. This includes your GP and the practice nurse who, in the first instance, will be able to assess the condition of the eczema, and also take a history of quality of life issues such as how much sleep is lost due to discomfort, scratching etc. This can afford the opportunity to change some of the skin treatment currently being used and try alternative creams and ointments. Trying more intensive skin routines for a short period can often help you through a difficult phase. Also ask for any information regarding local support groups; sometimes health centres run support groups for eczema sufferers. Your GP will also be able to provide advice about other health professionals available for referral, such as clinical psychologists who are trained to help people with chronic conditions who require extra support. It is possible to learn ways of thinking about and responding to various problems, such as chronic disease, that make them easier to bear – these are called 'coping mechanisms'.

## STRESS

**Does stress make eczema worse? My daughter tends to get wound up about things and I notice her scratching a lot more.**

Stress and other types of emotional arousal can certainly make eczema worse, and children with eczema do seem prone to stress. Some common emotions that contribute to this are anger, anxiety, sadness and feelings of guilt, and all of these can be related to having itchy red skin. The emotional stress tends to lead to increased sweating, which irritates the skin and triggers itching so the eczema gets worse. Children can get trapped in a vicious circle in which they worry about having eczema, sweat, feel more itchy and worry even more. You need to explore your daughter's feelings, perhaps with the help of a nurse, counsellor or one of her teachers, and find ways to help her relax. Some counsellors are skilled in teaching relaxation techniques and some hospital physiotherapy departments may be able to help by training your daughter in special ways of breathing to help her relax. Your doctor should know if this is available in your area. Other ways of relaxing can be taught or used by complementary practitioners (see Chapter 6).

### Is there a connection between hyperactivity and eczema?

This is a difficult question to answer accurately as it hasn't been well studied. Psychological factors are certainly important in eczema. Children who get stressed or upset may scratch more and worsen their eczema, but the role of hyperactivity is less clear. In general, children with eczema are more likely to be introverted than extroverted. A point to consider is that antihistamines used in eczema can occasionally cause stimulation and hyperactivity rather than the usual response of sedation. If this is the case, the antihistamine should be changed or stopped. There is certainly no evidence that eczema causes hyperactivity.

## PETS

**My daughter is very attached to our rather elderly family cat, but I have noticed that she scratches furiously after spending any length of time stroking her. I know that having pets is not recommended when you have eczema but I am reluctant to get rid of the cat. What should I do?**

Unfortunately, pets are not a good idea with eczema but you have to balance the psychological implications of getting rid of the cat with the benefits. The problem with cats is not with the fur itself but with a protein in the saliva, and you only have to watch a cat washing to realise that this is all over it. Where possible, try to limit the cat to a few rooms in the house, banning it from the bedrooms and areas where you normally carry out skin treatment. Wearing cotton gloves may allow your daughter to stroke the cat without too much irritation. Other sensible precautions are:

- never allow pets on or under the bed;
- do not allow pets near any bed linen;
- put down a cotton sheet when children play on the carpet to prevent their coming into contact with carpet fibres and animal hairs.

When the cat dies you may have to be very firm and resist the temptation to replace her. Avoiding fur, hair and feathers may mean you have to opt for a goldfish!

## SOFT TOYS

**My son is very attached to his teddy. Should I try to swap it for something less irritant for his eczema?**

If your son is 'very attached' to his teddy, this will probably be very difficult. Soft toys can be a problem for children with eczema as they harbour the house dust mite, but, as mentioned earlier (Chapter 4), the exact role of the house dust

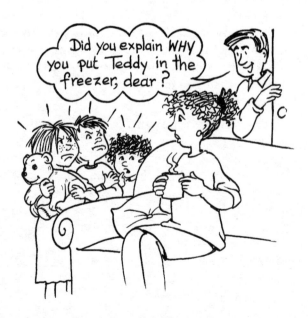

mite in making eczema worse is not clear. Ideally, all stuffed toys should be avoided but this can be very difficult indeed. If children do have soft toys, the following measures will be helpful in reducing any effect from the house dust mite.

- If possible, wash the teddy at a temperature higher than 55°C.
- Some toys cannot withstand these temperatures, so put them in a plastic bag and freeze for six hours to kill any house dust mites and then wash according to the manufacturer's instructions.
- Try to get two or three of your son's favourite soft toy so that he always has one while the other is in the freezer or the wash.
- Hang the teddy outside on the line when it's sunny – the sun kills house dust mites.

## HOUSEWORK

**Having a toddler with eczema running around, I find it very difficult to know the best time to tackle the housework.**

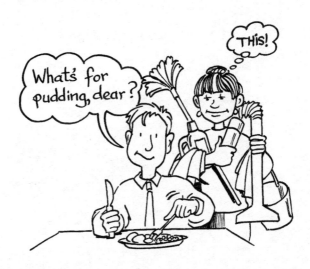

With young children – and especially one with eczema – developing a good routine is usually quite helpful, considering the amount of time involved in cleaning and general housework. It is better to carry out vacuuming and dusting when your child has an afternoon nap or perhaps in the evening when you could get your partner to help. Vacuuming disturbs the house dust mites in the soft furnishings, and this could be irritant to the child's skin. Damp dusting is more beneficial than using polish, especially in your child's bedroom.

# CHAPTER 8

## *School*

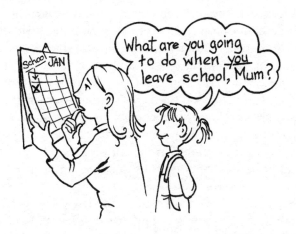

School plays a major part in children's lives but, sadly for those with eczema, starting school can be the first time they can feel 'different' and come up against teasing, bullying and prejudice. Many people still see eczema and other skin diseases as being 'infectious' or due to a lack of hygiene. You may also find that you can have as many problems as your child because of adverse comments from other parents.

## INFORMING THE SCHOOL

**Do I need to tell the school about my daughter's eczema?**

No, you do not 'need' to but you will probably find that she has many fewer problems if you have a discussion about eczema with her teachers. They can then be on the look-out for problems such as teasing and bullying, and will be aware of the problems some activities at school might cause – and how to overcome them. You can also take the opportunity to ensure that the school understands eczema and correct any mistaken beliefs.

**Should the school or my son keep his creams when he is at school?**

Without knowing more details about your son, this is a difficult question to answer. Most of the 'active' treatments for eczema (i.e. topical steroids and tablets) are used only once or twice a day, so should not need to be given at school. The only exception to this is some of the antibiotics. This leaves your son's moisturiser and soap substitute as the only creams that he will usually need at school. You should find out the school's policy and make sure it allows for easy access to the creams for washing his hands. Most schools will keep prescription drugs that need to be given regularly but should have a more flexible policy towards creams, as they tend to have with asthma inhalers. You need to make sure that your son is happy and confident about using his creams and that he can have some privacy at school when he feels the need to apply them.

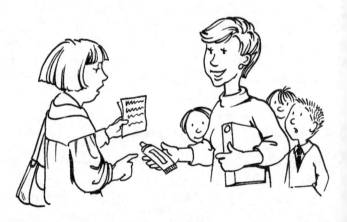

**My son has a very bad habit of scratching when he's bored and left to his own devices. What will happen at school if the teacher doesn't notice him?**

You need to discuss your concerns with your son's teacher. You may well find that he is usually so absorbed in activities at school that he doesn't have time, or forgets, to scratch. It would be worth suggesting that he sits somewhere in the classroom away from a sunny window, radiator or other source of heat so that he doesn't feel itchy from being too hot. Make sure that some moisturiser is readily available to soothe his skin if he becomes itchy and that he has time to apply it. Don't fall into the trap of getting the teacher to stop him scratching by telling him off – this type of negative feedback will do more harm than good.

# COPING WITH IRRITATION

**My son's hands are constantly exposed to water, paints and sand in the nursery he attends. Is there anything I can do to minimise the damage caused by these?**

Water play is common and problems with this can be overcome by asking the teacher to add to the water some of the bath oil your child normally uses. This can prevent dryness and soreness in your child's hands. Also make sure that there is a supply of your child's particular soap substitute available to use, as soaps and detergent will irritate the skin. With 'dry' activities such as painting and sand play, your son might be able to wear cotton gloves to provide some protection to his hands. Fine cotton gloves are available from chemists and can be prescribed. Ask your GP to provide smaller tubes of moisturising creams that you can leave at the school, or decant some into small tubs to be used two or three times during the day when possible.

**My daughter loves reading and writing but sometimes the eczema on her hands is so bad she can't hold a pen.**

Learning to write will be difficult with sore, cracked, dry fingers. Carrying out more intensive skin treatment during this phase will improve the skin. Also, wearing cotton gloves following the application of creams will enhance the treatment and prevent further damage. Discuss with her teacher the possibility of waiting for a couple of days before resuming writing activities, or see if using a computer would be an acceptable alternative as she could still practise spelling and sentence creation with a simple word-processing package.

**I find it very difficult to deal with my 5-year-old son's eczema now that he has started full-time school. Lots of his school 'play' activities include things that seem to make his eczema worse or at the least difficult to manage.**

Starting full-time school is an exciting prospect for most children but it can cause some problems for children with eczema. It is important to establish a good line of communication with the school staff. Making a special appointment with the staff to discuss openly your son's eczema and your particular concerns and anxieties beforehand would be worth while. Ideally, a pot of emollient cream should be kept at school, clearly labelled with your son's name and directions for use to be applied as necessary. Steroid creams and ointments are best kept for use at home only.

Emphasise to school staff and other parents that eczema is not contagious; however, make sure that teachers are aware that your son should avoid skin-to-skin contact with anyone who has a cold sore, as this can lead to eczema herpeticum. The National Eczema Society produce a good booklet for teachers on *Eczema in School*, and it is well worth giving your school a copy.

## SWIMMING AND SPORT

**Should I allow my son to go swimming with his class? I'm worried that it may make his eczema worse but it's his favourite activity and I don't want to say no to him.**

Swimming can be troublesome for children with eczema

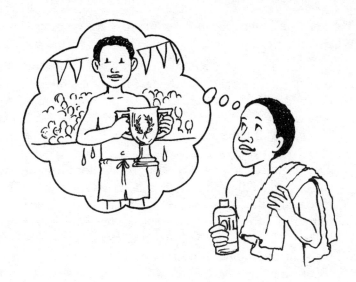

and school swimming sessions can pose their own particular problems. Showers afterwards tend to be mayhem
with a class of children but the teacher may be willing to
ensure that he at least applies moisturiser before dressing.
Follow this up with a good oily bath when he returns home
and plenty of moisturiser to counteract the drying effect of
the chlorine in the swimming pool. Swimming should be
encouraged, and not prohibited simply because of eczema,
as it is often fun and is part of **normal** life. An emollient can
also be used before swimming, with very greasy preparations such as emulsifying ointment or paraffin mixtures
being applied to protect areas of cracked skin. The only
concern with this approach is that it will make his skin
slippery, which is a disadvantage if someone tries to help
him out of the pool.

If your son's eczema is very active or infected, however, it
would be best if he stopped swimming for a short time. This
is both because his skin will be much more prone to irritation and also to avoid the possibility of his feeling
embarrassed at getting undressed (see Chapter 9).

**My son won't take part in PE at school because of his eczema. What can we do?**

It is important to sit down and talk to your son to find out why he doesn't like doing PE. Some children simply don't like PE, but it may be that he is worried about what his classmates will say if they see the eczema on his skin. He may well have experienced some teasing, name-calling or even bullying. If this is the case, arrange to see his teacher to discuss the problem. If children usually wear shorts and singlets in PE, the school may well be prepared to change the rules and let children wear tracksuit bottoms and sweatshirts. This simple measure has certainly helped with a number of our children. PE may also make his skin feel itchy as he gets hot, and you may have to ensure that he can cool down with a shower afterwards and apply his moisturiser.

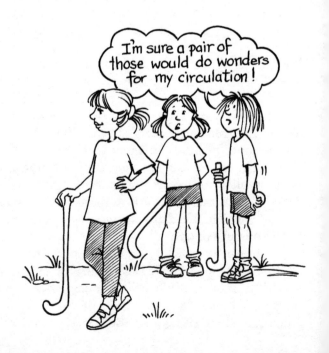

**I'm worried that my daughter may be teased at school because of her eczema, as it is usually very bad on her legs and I'm not sure how she will cope with sports.**

Teasing and bullying do exist and can be very difficult to cope with. Be alert to any problems that may arise and discuss them with the teacher. Asking your daughter how she is coping is a good starting point, and she may be able to express any anxieties and be willing to talk about them. Most schools have a policy to deal with bullying.

As far as sports are concerned, have a word with the teacher responsible to discuss whether it would be possible for her to wear cotton leggings instead of shorts if she is embarrassed about the state of the eczema on her legs. Most schools are co-operative in this type of situation.

# STATEMENT OF SPECIAL EDUCATIONAL NEEDS

**I have recently visited the school my child is due to start this year to explain about her eczema, which is severe. They have suggested that I apply to have her 'statemented'. What does this mean and how do I go about it?**

The 1981 Education Act stated that all children should, wherever possible, be integrated into mainstream schools. This was the start of 'statements of special educational needs', in which, where necessary, a statement is prepared of a child's educational needs and the extra support that should be provided in the school.

We would advise any parent of a child with special needs to find out as much as possible about 'statements' from their local education authority, and to use it to get the best for their child. The age of your child does not matter, as you do not have to wait until your child is old enough to go to school before starting the statementing process. The Department for Education and Employment publishes a booklet called *Special Educational Needs – A Guide for Parents* (see Appendix 2), which outlines the procedures and explains the jargon used. Most people think of 'special educational needs' as relating only to children with learning difficulties but it applies equally to children with severe physical problems, and unfortunately eczema can fall into this category. We recommend that you seek help with your application from a body such as the National Eczema Society.

# SPECIALIST SCHOOLS

**Are there special schools for children with eczema?**

A special boarding school did exist for children with very severe eczema and/or severe asthma. This was The Pilgrim's School in East Sussex. The staff at Pilgrim's were skilled and experienced in dealing with eczema, and children had easy access to nurses, physiotherapists and psychologists. Sadly, the school closed at Christmas 1997 because of funding problems and we don't know of any other such school.

# EXAMS

**My son has to sit exams this summer. He has not missed any school but I am worried that his eczema may interfere with these exams. Is there anything I can do to help him?**

The first thing to mention is that research studies have shown that most children with eczema perform at school as well as those without eczema. Having said that, the stress of exams combined with hot summer weather can sometimes cause eczema to flare up. Make sure that your son has a cool shady room to revise in. If he does his own treatments, try to discuss with him a plan of action **he** would like to adopt if the eczema does flare. Ask if he is happy with his creams – or does he find them too greasy? Lighter creams are often better during the summer. Intensifying topical therapy is the best approach for flare-ups. Try to avoid systemic treatments such as oral steroids or antihistamines, which may interfere with sleep patterns or concentration.

If he does have a bad flare-up that you and he feel has prevented him from producing his best work in an exam, discuss this with his tutor. You may be able to get the examining board to take this into consideration. They will usually require a confirming letter from his doctor, so if he does have a flare-up it is worth taking him to your doctor even if you can alter his treatment yourself to cope with it. A doctor cannot write a letter saying your son's eczema has been a problem if he or she didn't see him at the time.

# CHAPTER 9

## Social life and holidays

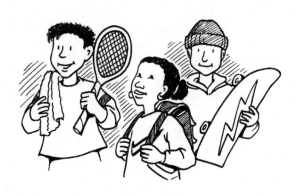

This chapter inevitably has some overlap with other chap‑
ters but allows us to include problems related to social life
such as make-up and hairstyles. It also looks at some of the
problems that children with more severe eczema can have
when going on holiday.

## SPORT

**Why does my son feel itchy after playing football?**

Any sport or activity that leads to sweating can cause
itching. Indoor sports, such as karate, five-a-side football,
squash and badminton, tend to be worse than outdoor
sports because the sweat doesn't evaporate as quickly as
when out of doors. Sweat itself is very irritant. Think of the
stinging that sweat causes if it drips in your eye. Sweat has
exactly the same irritant effect on the sensitive skin of
eczema. Having said that, your son, like all children with

eczema, should still be encouraged to engage in sporting activities, as they are part of normal life. If he does become itchy after football, he should try a luke-warm shower and an application of moisturiser.

**Can I take my baby swimming even though she has eczema?**

Yes, children with eczema should be encouraged to learn to swim, but chlorinated swimming pools do have a tendency to dry and irritate the skin. You can make this less of a problem by the following approach:

- apply a moisturiser before swimming;
- shower after swimming to remove the chlorine;
- reapply some moisturiser.

It may be worth avoiding swimming during bad flare-ups of eczema. The water may make things worse, and we have heard of children being asked, quite unreasonably, by pool attendants not to swim because they think 'it is catching'. This is not true but just reflects ignorance and distresses the child and parent. Whilst we applaud parents fighting against this intolerance we are also aware of how such an experience can affect an older child's self-confidence so it may be better just to avoid such a situation. It is a fine balance between encouraging children with eczema to participate in everything and putting them in a difficult situation after which they might refuse to go swimming again.

   If swimming has to be avoided temporarily, it can be resumed as soon as the flare-up is controlled.

## MAKE-UP AND HAIRSTYLES

**My daughter wanted to have her face painted at a local fete. She has eczema but doesn't get it on her face. Is this OK?**

Yes, this would probably be OK. Whilst people can be

allergic to face paints, this is very rare – especially in children. If you were very concerned, you could always see what type of paint they use and apply some to a forearm for a couple of days first to make sure there was no reaction and then allow her to have her face painted next time.

However, if your daughter has very bad facial eczema, it would probably be sensible to avoid face paints as they can cause irritation. A good mask or costume might provide an alternative and remove any disappointment for your daughter.

### Is it all right for my 14-year-old girl to wear make-up?

Yes; provided the eczema is reasonably controlled, this is acceptable. Every effort should be made to treat children with eczema the same as other children. It would be worth trying out the make-up on a forearm for a few days to check that there is no adverse reaction. If it is OK, the make-up can be used elsewhere. It is advisable to use one of the hypoallergenic make-ups, such as those by ROC and Clinique, who have always made good cosmetic products. Remember, though, that even these can cause irritation or allergic problems at times.

If your daughter's eczema has a bad flare-up and there is weepy, broken skin, it would be advisable to avoid make-up for a while.

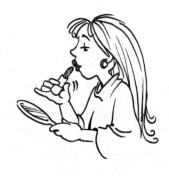

**My son wants to have his hair cut very short, as it seems to be the in thing at his school. Will this affect his eczema?**

No, it's unlikely to have any impact on his eczema, even if his scalp is affected – and it is important for your son to fit in with current fashion. Very short hair and head shaving are done for both religious and fashion reasons, but we have not seen either of these cause any problem with eczema.

**My daughter has eczema. Should I allow her to get her ears pierced?**

Yes; provided she doesn't have active eczema of her ears, this is fine. Some parents worry that children with eczema will go on to develop nickel allergy from the earrings but in fact this is no more common in people with atopic eczema than in those without. Even if nickel allergy does develop, there are a number of metals that do not contain nickel – for example, good quality gold, British sterling silver and platinum. Earrings probably cause problems because the residue of soap and shampoo can build up around them, leading to an irritant eczema, so they should be removed before hair washing, showering or bathing.

**My daughter has typical African/Caribbean hair and wants to straighten it. What should I advise her?**

Hair straightening is popular in African/Caribbean people and we would not want your daughter to stand out as being different from her friends. There are three different techniques that can achieve this: heat, acid and alkali – the two chemical 'relaxers' used with the second and third methods are more common today. They all act by breaking the disulphide chemical bonds in the hair that make it naturally curly.

- **Heat**  Combing with hot oils was popular but has rather gone out of fashion recently because it has to be repeated more frequently.

- **Acid**  This uses an acid chemical called ammonium thioglycolate, also used in perms.
- **Alkali**  The chemical used here is sodium hydroxide (an alkali).

Both chemical methods also have to use neutralising chemicals to stop the reaction. If the chemicals are left on too long, they will cause a chemical burn of the scalp, so it is important to find an experienced hairdresser for straightening to ensure that the chemicals are used correctly.

All the above methods can be irritant to broken skin and we do not feel that one technique is better than another with regard to eczema. If your daughter has eczema of the scalp, she should avoid hair straightening until her eczema has completely resolved. Fortunately, eczema of the scalp is relatively rare in older children, and eczema elsewhere on the body should not stop her from having it done.

## COMPUTERS

**My child spends a lot of time playing at his computer. Could this be affecting his eczema?**

No, there is no evidence that electrical equipment, such as computers, affects eczema. If his hands are occupied playing a computer game, he will probably not be scratching – so sitting at a computer may be better than sitting watching television with nothing to keep his hands busy.

## VISITING FRIENDS

**My 4-year-old daughter has recently been invited to a friend's birthday party. She is on a dairy-free diet for her eczema. How can I be sure she won't be given any dairy products?**

It is difficult to be completely sure but speak to her friend's parents to see if they are prepared to help. Remember, though, that to have completely separate food may make your daughter feel different or singled out. Don't be too worried, because, even if she does have an occasional break from her diet, it is unlikely to cause any problem. In any case, exclusion diets tend to be more beneficial in children younger than she is, so a lapse in your daughter's diet is unlikely to have a major impact on her eczema. If she has been on the diet for some time, it is probably worth trying her on dairy products again as her hypersensitivity may have reduced. Any re-introduction of food must be done **slowly** and in small amounts over a few months.

However, in cases of allergy to substances such as eggs or nuts, producing swelling of the lips, wheezing and fainting, these foods **MUST be avoided COMPLETELY** at all times (see Chapter 4).

# HOLIDAYS

**Is there a mosquito repellent suitable for children with eczema?**

The 'physical' methods are preferable to the chemical methods: i.e. the use of appropriate clothing, long-sleeved cotton shirts and long trousers, and a mosquito net at night. All these should be used in addition to any other form of repellent if possible.

Mosquito coils and burners can also be useful at night if a net isn't available, but perhaps the best 'non-contact' device is a plug-in repellent that works off an electric socket. All of the mosquito repellents put directly onto the skin can cause some irritation if the eczema is active. The liquid ones are usually alcohol based and may cause stinging. If you are still keen to use one, try applying it to a test-area on a forearm for a few days before you go away, to check that it doesn't cause any irritation, before using it on larger areas.

**I want to go on holiday but am worried about going to a hotel where things in the environment might make my child's eczema worse. Can you advise?**

Holidays should be a time for everybody in the family to relax, and most children find that their eczema improves on holidays – probably due to a combination of sunshine, relaxation and change of environment. You will have to be a little careful in choosing the environment, based on your knowledge of what tends to make your child's eczema worse. Checking ahead is vital because you should try to avoid old, traditional hotels that may have deep-pile carpets and heavy curtains to harbour house dust mite (HDM). Feather duvets and pillows may also be a problem, and many parents carry a cotton sleeping-bag liner if they are concerned about bedding. Extremes of air-conditioning and central heating can be a problem but most hotels allow you to turn them down if needed. You can't, however, alter outside temperatures and hot, humid conditions can be very uncomfortable for someone with eczema.

Over all, seaside holidays seem to be best for children with eczema, although sand can be an irritant. But remember not to be seen to choose the holiday for this reason only, if other family members would prefer a different holiday, as this could cause tension in your family.

Finally, remember to take enough treatment on holiday with you – extra moisturiser is often needed and can be difficult to obtain overseas. If you are flying, pack some

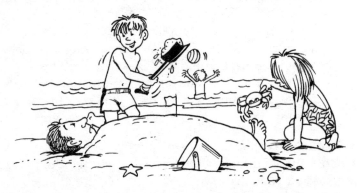

cream in your hand luggage in case you are delayed or your suitcases get lost!

**We are about to go on holiday in Spain. My son suffers with bad eczema. Should we be worried about the strong sunshine, and can you recommend any suitable sunblock creams?**

He may find that his eczema improves on a sunny holiday, provided the weather isn't too hot. This may be due in part to the ultraviolet rays in the sunshine, which are recognised as damping down inflammation in the skin. (We occasionally use artificial ultraviolet therapy to treat very bad eczema in children – see Chapter 5.)

However, one must remember that too much sunshine is bad for the skin and may increase the risk of skin cancer in later life. If your son has skin that never tans but just burns, he should avoid the sun as much as possible. Long-sleeved cotton shirts, sun hats and sun blocks should be encouraged. If he does tan, some gentle sun exposure can be encouraged but make sure he **never** burns. Start the holiday with only a little exposure and build up gently. Avoid the middle of the day when the sun is at its most fierce. Even Asian or African/Caribbean children can occasionally burn, although obviously the risks are much smaller.

A large number of sunblock creams are available today to protect you when out in the sun, but they should not be used as a way of staying out longer because they don't give complete protection. Any product that has a sun protection factor (SPF) of 15 or above is suitable. There is actually very little difference between these factor numbers once you have reached factor 15 or above. The product should also say that it protects against UVB and UVA light. We do not like the term 'total' sun block – even a completely opaque cream will rub off and lose effectiveness.

Sunblocks come in two types: chemical absorbers or reflectors. The reflectors are less likely to cause an allergic problem but they are not as cosmetically acceptable for some people because they cause a rather opaque white appearance. We don't have strong views as to which is better but it is important to find a sunblock that your son is prepared to use. Some sunblocks are said to be water-proof but 'water-resistant' might be a better description, as swimming will decrease their effectiveness to some degree and they will need to be reapplied.

When you have chosen a sunblock cream, use it twice daily on a test area on the arm to check that there is no adverse irritation. Do this for a few days before you go on holiday in case you have to find another. Remember that the best and the cheapest sunblock, which doesn't have to be reapplied, is good-quality cotton clothing. A final point to remember is that sunshine is drying to the skin, so your son may need to use more moisturiser, or a greasier one, than normal.

**Our son wants to go on scout camp. He has had bad eczema for some years and we are worried about his treatments. Should we stop him from going?**

If your son is old enough to go on scout camp, he should be old enough to apply his own treatments and may already be doing so. As children with eczema grow up, they should be encouraged to become more independent and to start doing their own treatments. In view of this we think that it is important for you to allow your son to go on scout camp. It would be worth having a word with the camp organisers in advance, letting them know about your son's condition and how it should be treated – everybody will have to fill in a medical form. They may well have dealt with similar situations before, bearing in mind how common eczema has become. If you are still concerned, you could always arrange for an organiser to phone you during the camp to let you know that all is well.

**Are there any special holidays available for children with eczema?**

Yes, there is a programme called Peak (formerly the Joint Holiday Project). This has been set up jointly by the National Eczema Society and the National Asthma Campaign. It is aimed at people with eczema, asthma or both. Holidays are arranged in different areas within the UK during the summer months, aimed at providing a safe, happy and active environment for children to help build up their confidence. Holidays are provided for different age groups, including teenagers. A variety of activities, especially sport, are encouraged. The holidays are run by a mixture of parents, medical personnel and staff from the National Eczema Society and the National Asthma Campaign. Similar holidays are run in the USA if your child is feeling more adventurous and would like to go further afield (see Appendix 1).

**Since we booked our package holiday, we have been told by a friend that her child had problems joining in with the activities organised by the holiday reps for children. Will this be a problem?**

It all depends on the severity of your child's eczema, the reaction of the individual holiday rep and the activities involved. The representative may be subject to a company policy or be allowed to make his or her own judgements. Try to find out more about the company's approach before you go, and seek out your holiday rep to explain that eczema is not catching etc., when you get to the resort.

**Do I need to declare my daughter's eczema when arranging travel insurance?**

Without knowing the details of the application form, it is difficult to say anything other than 'probably'. It will be regarded as a **pre-existing condition** so, if not mentioned, might be excluded from the cover.

### Can we get access to medical care abroad?

This depends on which country you visit, but your travel agent or holiday company should be able to advise you. Medical attention is free in all European Community countries as long as you have certificate **E111**, available from the Post Office. The Department of Health produces a booklet called *The Traveller's Guide to Health*.

# CHAPTER 10

## Growing up

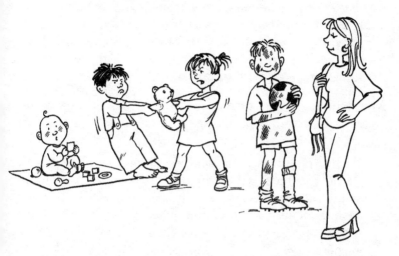

Children with eczema grow up and, although many will grow out of their eczema, it will continue to be a problem for some of them throughout their teenage years. Others grow out of atopic eczema but may develop more of an irritant pattern of eczema, especially on the hands. This chapter deals with some aspects that apply to children at different stages of childhood, although there is much overlap with other chapters in the book.

## IMMUNISATION

**Are there any immunisations my baby should avoid?**

No, all immunisations should be given normally to children with eczema. As with other children, your doctor might delay the immunisations if your baby is suffering from an acute illness or has a raised temperature. A flare-up of eczema without general illness is not a reason for delay.

Some children are still offered a BCG (Bacille Calmette–Guérin) vaccination to protect against tuberculosis. Although this is no longer routine, it is given when there is a high risk of exposure to tuberculosis. This includes people in inner city areas, children whose families have come from high-risk countries (such as India and Pakistan) and contacts of cases of tuberculosis. The only precaution to take when giving BCG is to use normal skin for the injection site rather than skin with eczema.

**My child has both eczema and asthma, so he uses steroid creams and steroid inhalers. Isn't it dangerous for him to have immunisations?**

No, the only reason for delaying immunisation because of steroid treatment is if the steroids are being given by mouth as tablets or medicine. Usually the child will be too ill to have immunisations but, even when the course of steroids has finished, you should wait three months before the injections.

Children (and adults) with asthma should have an injection against influenza each year. This vaccine is prepared in eggs, so should not be given to anyone who is allergic to them. If you feel that eggs have made your son's eczema or asthma worse, he can have a skin-prick test to check this (see Chapter 2). Even if he **is** allergic to eggs, it may be possible for him to have the injection under the supervision of a community paediatrician via your GP.

## SHAVING

**My teenage son gets eczema on his face and has recently started to shave. Which is the best shaving method?**

This is a difficult question to answer, as some people have problems with both wet and dry (electric) shaving. Irritation can arise from the physical trauma of shaving and also from the various shaving products used. It is best to use

**unscented** products, which will usually be labelled 'For Sensitive Skin'. Your son may have to experiment a bit. If he would like to wet shave, it is important that he gets a good quality razor – for example, one that is guarded by a wire mesh to prevent cuts – and changes the blades regularly.

For wet shaving he should try the following.

- Apply a thick layer of moisturiser to the beard area and allow it to soak in; this can take a few minutes.
- Wet the face thoroughly.
- Apply a generous amount of shaving gel or foam, or even use more moisturiser as a 'shaving gel'.
- Shave in the direction of hair growth, i.e. the direction in which the skin feels smoother. This will generally be downwards on the face but may be in several different directions, especially on the neck.
- Rinse and dry.
- Apply some more moisturiser.

Shaving in the direction of the hair growth will leave the hair a little longer than shaving against the growth. Having a very close shave can cause more damage to the skin. It can also cause problems in African/Caribbeans, and others with curly hair, as the curled hair tends to grow back into the skin, causing inflamed lumps that can get infected. If your son would like to try a closer shave, he could shave against the hair growth after shaving with the growth and after a further application of foam, gel or moisturiser.

For dry shaving, your son should get a good quality electric razor. It is worth applying moisturiser before and after, but a longer time is needed before shaving to allow the moisturiser to soak in thoroughly so that the grease doesn't clog the razor.

After-shaves can cause problems because they contain alcohol and can cause stinging and drying. If your son wants to use one, he should use a minimal amount and avoid any areas of irritated skin.

**Moisturisers are a bone of contention in our house. My teenager says he doesn't like the ones he has been prescribed and wants to use ones he buys himself. Should I allow him to do this?**

Yes, is the simple answer – at least he is willing to use moisturisers. It is a very welcome fact that there are lots of moisturisers and skin care products for men these days, and many companies produce very good ones. Makes such as Clinique, Body Shop and Boots own-brand range offer 'hypoallergenic' or 'sensitive skin' products that are usually suitable for people with eczema. They can be expensive but we'll leave the discussion about who pays to you and your son!

## CAREERS ADVICE

**My daughter has set her heart on being a nurse but she had eczema as a child. Is this likely to stop her from getting a job?**

No, your daughter can still get a job as a nurse but the following must be considered and discussed sympathetically with her. As a nurse, she will undoubtedly be at increased risk of developing eczema again, especially of the hands. This is particularly true if she had troublesome hand eczema as a child, even if the eczema has been gone for many years. Nursing inevitably entails frequent washing of the hands, which can cause irritation to the skin and make a recurrence of eczema more likely. If the eczema does come back during her nursing, it may significantly interfere with the job. Although using gloves to protect the skin, using aqueous cream as a soap substitute for washing and using a hand moisturising cream regularly may help, these measures may not be sufficient to stop her developing bad eczema.

We are sorry to say that we have seen some nurses who

have had to give up their chosen profession because of troublesome eczema. This seems a terrible waste after many years of dedication and training, so we would advise you to have a long chat with your daughter explaining the risks and even arrange for her to talk it through with a nurse. You may mention that there are many other worthwhile jobs in health care such as physiotherapy, occupational health, management etc., which will have much less risk of provoking a recurrence of her eczema.

**My child has just seen a careers adviser at school. She has had bad eczema since she was a baby. Are there any careers she should avoid?**

This is a very important consideration for your daughter, especially as she still has troublesome eczema. There are a number of careers that can make eczema worse or cause a recurrence of eczema in people who have grown out of it. Jobs that involve manual work and frequent contact with irritants are the least desirable. The following might cause problems:

- hairdressing,
- catering/food handling,

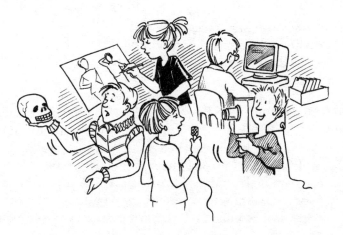

- nursing,
- floristry/gardening,
- engineering/garage mechanic,
- animal handling/vet/veterinary nurse,
- building/working with cement,
- the armed forces (medical entrance requirements may be difficult).

We feel it is important that you sit down with your daughter at an early stage to explain the situation and see how she feels. It can be helpful to take the view that horizons are changed, not necessarily narrowed. It is better to deal with this possible problem at an early stage rather than after she is committed to a chosen career and has started the training. In general, non-manual jobs – such as administration, computer-based work, journalism, film making, singing, fashion design, teaching or any office-based work – are the most suitable. If she seems uninterested, try to arrange for any friends in appropriate jobs to show her around their workplace. Take the opportunity of any work experience schemes available through her school. Other people she could talk to about her career include:

- doctor or skin specialist;
- university career advisory service;
- the disablement employment adviser (contact your local JobCentre).

### My son is about to leave school and still has eczema. Will he have to tell future employers about his skin?

Yes; he is legally obliged to tell employers about any medical condition, including eczema. An employer, or their occupational health department, may ask for further details to try to assess how severe the condition has been. In general, it is unlikely that having eczema would decrease your son's chances of obtaining most jobs – with the exception of those mentioned in the previous answer.

# RELATIONSHIPS

**My daughter is 15 and most of her friends have boyfriends. I am sure she would have a boyfriend but for her eczema. She won't talk about it to me or my husband. What can we do to help her?**

This is a difficult problem but there are probably a number of factors involved. We do not know how bad your daughter's eczema is, but, even if mild, it is likely to affect her at this age. It is difficult enough at the best of times for children to deal with a changing body and emotions, and any minor blemishes such as warts or spots can assume great importance. If she has eczema on visible areas such as the hands or face this can be devastating to her self-confidence.

Teenagers are frequently reluctant to talk to their parents. They often feel unloved and unwanted and may blame their eczema as the sole cause of their problems. Your daughter may have become disillusioned and fed up with treatment and is now using it less often. She may find some of the ointments too greasy and cosmetically unacceptable. Teenage years can be very trying times for both child and parents! There is no easy approach to this problem. If your daughter has a close family friend or relative whom she confides in, it may be worth enlisting their support. Also your doctor or specialist may be able to provide a sympathetic ear for her. A review of her treatment would be worthwhile anyway to try to find something that suits her and that she is prepared to use.

Finally, the National Eczema Society may be able to put her in touch locally with other children of the same age who have the same problems. She may be able to express herself more easily with them than with her parents. These measures may help build up her self-confidence, but, although you can facilitate this, she must be allowed to find her own feet at her own pace.

# SEX, PERIODS AND PREGNANCY

**Would it be dangerous to become pregnant while on eczema medication?**

If the treatment is just topical creams, the answer would be no – even though the steroid preparations tend to carry a warning about pregnancy. The systemic therapies, prednisolone, cyclosporin and azathioprine, and PUVA therapy **must** be avoided throughout pregnancy. **All** tablets should be avoided for the first three months of pregnancy if at all possible. If antibiotics **have** to be given, penicillin and erythromycin are suitable. Antihistamines can usually be avoided in pregnancy but are thought to be safe. Chlorpheniramine (Piriton) is often used and is regarded as one of the safest.

If eczema herpeticum develops, oral aciclovir is recommended because it seems to be relatively safe and any risk is far less serious than leaving the condition untreated.

**My daughter has recently asked me for some advice about contraception. Will her eczema cause any complications?**

It is very unlikely that she will have problems with any form of contraception. Although latex (rubber) allergy may occur in adults, causing problems with condoms and the cap, it is extremely rare in children and young adults. Latex allergy is seen occasionally in children who have had frequent surgical operations involving the insertion of latex shunts or catheters, but if your daughter has not had such treatment there should be no problem.

**My daughter has recently started having periods and finds that her eczema gets worse before each monthly bleed. What can she do about this?**

Hormones can have an effect on eczema and this can be an extra problem on top of all the other changes related to puberty. We are afraid that this area is poorly understood. What she can do depends on how bad the flare-up is and how old she is. It would be sensible to try simple treatment measures first – making the best use of soap substitutes and moisturisers – and then considering using a topical steroid more frequently or in a stronger form.

If the pre-menstrual flare-up is very severe, 'hormonal manipulation' might help but this is still a controversial treatment and the way it works is not yet clear. Treatment might include the contraceptive pill, but this carries some risks, so you would need to consider carefully the risks and benefits with your doctor.

# COPING WITH ACNE

**My teenage son still has eczema and has begun to develop acne. Does he need to change his eczema treatment?**

This is a tricky problem for him and he is unlucky, as it is somewhat unusual for acne and eczema to occur together. The type of eczema that causes most problems on the face is seborrhoeic eczema but atopic eczema also occurs here. It is difficult to imagine how skin can be both dry with eczema and greasy with acne but they can happen on different parts of the face. His eczema treatment on the face should be no more than a moisturiser and occasional mild topical steroid. A light moisturiser is advisable to try to prevent clogging of pores.

If he uses a topical treatment for his acne, he could have problems because many of the preparations contain alcohol or other substances that can dry the skin. Your doctor can discuss how to use tablet treatment, which could manage his acne adequately without making the eczema worse.

# MISCELLANEOUS

**Will my child grow out of her eczema?**

There is a good chance that your child's eczema will improve or disappear altogether with time. It is difficult to predict accurately when this will happen but about 50% of children with early-onset eczema (it starts before the age of one year) will have improved significantly by the age of five; more than 90% will have improved by the age of 18. However, if the onset of eczema was later in childhood, especially if it appeared in teenage years, the outlook is not as good.

**My 15-year-old daughter has had eczema affecting her elbows and knees for years. This has improved as she has got older but recently she has developed bad eczema around her eyes. Why is this?**

If her eczema is beginning to improve, it is unusual for it to suddenly appear at a previously unaffected site. It may well be that she has developed a genuine allergic eczema (contact eczema or contact dermatitis) around her eyes on top of her atopic eczema. The likeliest culprit is either eye make-up or nail varnish, as people frequently touch the skin around their eyes with their fingers. We would advise that your GP

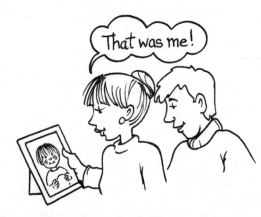

refer her to be patch-tested by your local dermatologist (see more about patch tests in Chapter 2).

**My son scratches his eczema until he bleeds. Will he be left with permanent scarring when he is older?**

We are happy to say this is unlikely. Even when someone seems to gouge out pieces of skin, it is amazing how well the skin recovers its normal state once the eczema has improved. Children with pigmented skin may, however, develop pigment changes, which can be unsightly and can last for many months or even years.

# CHAPTER 11

## Practical concerns

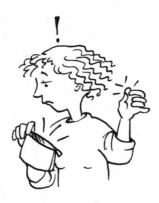

This chapter contains some practical advice about financial help and state benefits as well as the answers to some other questions that didn't seem to fit easily into other chapters.

## FINANCIAL CONSIDERATIONS

**Are there any benefits I am entitled to claim because my daughter has very bad eczema?**

Yes there are, but we would advise you to seek help with filling in the forms involved so that you can bring out the full impact that the eczema has on her life. For any benefit claim or financial worries we recommend that you seek assistance from your local Benefits Agency (part of the Department of Social Security) or see a hospital social worker. Sometimes the Citizens Advice Bureau can help with information.

**Disability Living Allowance (DLA)** is the first state benefit you should think about. This is not means-tested so your level of income will not affect the claim, and the allowance will not affect any other benefits you or your family may be claiming. When Disability Living Allowance is applied to children it reflects the care and help needed over and above what a healthy child would require, and is paid at different rates depending on the amount of help needed. More information and the current rates of the benefit are in leaflet **N1196**, 'Social Security Benefit Rates'. You can get the leaflet, along with the application packs, from any Benefits Agency office. A telephone help-line is also available: Benefit Enquiry Line – **0800 882 200** (a freephone number). The National Eczema Society can give advice about filling in the form.

For other benefits to which you might be entitled, see the next two questions.

**I spend a lot of time caring for my son and am unable to work. Can I get a benefit to help?**

If your son is in receipt of the middle or higher band of the Disabled Living Allowance, you may be able to claim **Invalid Care Allowance (ICA)** for yourself. You have to be spending at least 35 hours a week caring for your son and, as with Disabled Living Allowance mentioned above, this must be time you wouldn't have spent if he didn't have eczema. This benefit is also non-means-tested but you will have to declare it for tax purposes. The same Benefit Enquiry Line (**0800 88 22 00**) will give further information; you could also contact your local Citizens Advice Bureau (look in the telephone directory) or the Disability Alliance on 0171-247 8763 between 2.00 and 4.00 p.m. on Mondays and Wednesdays.

**I haven't been able to get any specific benefits and find it difficult to cope with the expense of special bedding and extra**

**laundry for my daughter with eczema. Is there any other way of getting help?**

If you are receiving any Social Security benefits, you may be able to get a loan or a grant from the Social Fund. Your local Benefits Agency office will give you more details.

There is also the Family Fund, an independent trust financed by the government. Grants are available to help families who are caring for a severely disabled child under 16. It is unlikely that a child who does not qualify for Disabled Living Allowance would be eligible but further information is available (see Appendix 2 for the address).

You could also consider the National Eczema Society's Welfare Fund, which is set up to help people with eczema and families on low income who have difficulty in meeting the cost of items such as cotton clothing, bedding and laundry services. Applications have to be made via a doctor, health visitor or social worker. For more information, apply to the National Eczema Society.

**My son will be 16 soon. As he is on four different preparations on prescription I am concerned about the cost – will he continue to get free prescriptions?**

If he is going on in full-time education to age 18, he will; if not, he won't. Costs of prescriptions can be a real problem for people with eczema because, unlike patients with epilepsy or diabetes, they are not entitled to free prescriptions. There is a current debate about the future of prescription charges but for now the only way of easing the burden if he has to pay is to buy a prepayment certificate. It's like a 'season ticket' for either three months or a whole year, and saves money if you need more than six prescriptions a quarter or 15 a year. Your pharmacist or doctor should be able to give you leaflet **FP95**, which explains how the scheme works.

# WASHING CLOTHES

**I have been told to change my washing powder to a non-biological one since my baby developed eczema, but which one should I use?**

Any non-biological washing powder is acceptable; there is no need to go to a great deal of expense. An efficient rinse and spin programme on your washing machine is essential. Research has shown that soap residue left on clothes from inefficient rinsing, handwashing or too much in one load of washing can be irritant to eczematous skin. (An extra rinse cycle with the washing machine can be helpful.) Fabric conditioners tend to be perfumed, so should be avoided. In hard water areas, water softeners can occasionally be beneficial.

**My daughter's clothes get very stained by her eczema treatment, especially the greasy moisturiser. How can I best wash them?**

Greasy ointments are particularly difficult to remove completely even during hot wash cycles. It is often best to use cream-based moisturisers during the day, where possible, as they cause less damage to clothing; greasy preparations can be used at bed-time when your daughter can wear old nightclothes. Biological washing powders are better than non-biological ones at removing grease and, provided the clothes are well rinsed, should not cause a problem with eczema.

**I have heard that grease can damage washing machines. Is this true?**

Yes, greasy moisturisers may cause the rubber seals on washing machines to age more quickly. These seals vary in quality, both between manufacturers and within model ranges. If you are thinking of buying a new machine, it is probably best to write to the manufacturers and ask for advice, as some seals are more resistant than others to this ageing.

We contacted Hotpoint, who gave us the following general advice. Once a month, carry out a 95°C wash with no clothes in the machine, using a biological powder because this helps to break down the grease and will unclog the system. If this is not your normal type of powder, do a second wash with your usual choice before washing your child's clothes.

# RESEARCH

**Are there going to be any breakthroughs in eczema treatment in the near future?**

We have to be realistic and say that a cure for eczema is not just around the corner. However, there are a number of areas of current research that may lead to better and safer therapies during the next decade.

We know that the body's immune system is in some way overactive in eczema and this drives the inflammation and itchiness in the skin. There are many researchers trying to find out which part of the immune system is responsible, thus paving the way for the development of new medications that will specifically inhibit this without affecting the rest of the immune system. We know that oral steroids are effective in eczema but they damp down most if not all the immune system and they have many side-effects. The relatively new drug **cyclosporin** is a more selective inhibitor but is still plagued by some unpleasant side-effects, especially as it has to be given by mouth. **Tacrolimus** is another selective immune-modifying drug, and has the advantage of being available in a topical form. This is currently under trial in atopic eczema and early results look encouraging. There is much interest around the world in new selective immune-modifying drugs, because they are potentially useful for so many medical conditions. There are a number of these drugs, which are currently under assessment. We predict that this area will produce newer, better and, hopefully, safer therapies in the near future.

You can't have failed to notice the huge explosion in genetic research over the last decade, with stories such as Dolly the cloned sheep making the headlines. This type of research has occurred in all areas of medicine, including dermatology. Many disorders caused by an abnormality in a single gene have now had the exact genetic mistake identified. However, as mentioned earlier, eczema has a very complicated inheritance and it is likely that many genes can be involved. Although three genetic areas of importance to atopic disease have been identified, we are still a long way from working out all the relevant genes.

Even when the genes have been identified, this does not give an instant treatment or cure. Gene therapy itself sounds like the perfect solution but this is still many years away even in single-gene conditions. Perhaps it will be more important to do further research into what the eczema genes do and what proteins they make. This would then give us some extra areas for designing specific new therapies.

Finally, an area that has received scant attention has been prevention and trigger factors. To prevent eczema rather than have to cure it is an attractive idea. Studies are currently looking at the role of newborns' diet, the importance of mothers breast-feeding and why certain racial groups have a higher incidence of eczema in certain countries or environments. Answers from these studies may give us scope to develop a more prevention-based approach to managing atopic eczema.

### How can I help with research into eczema?

If you would like to help from a financial viewpoint, there are a number of charities and skin research funds that provide money for scientists and dermatologists to embark on research projects into eczema. The best way to find out about these is to contact the National Eczema Society or the British Association of Dermatologists (addresses in Appendix 1). We should also mention that the National Eczema Society and the British Association of Dermatologists are involved with the All Party Parliamentary Group on Skin. This Group is very useful as it helps inform Parliament about the amount of skin disease in the UK and the impact it has on individuals and their families. It acts as a useful lobbying group when it comes to allocating medical resources for dermatology research, care and training.

If you are interested in finding out about new trials in eczema treatment, again the National Eczema Society and the British Association of Dermatologists will give you up-to-date information about these and, if interested, how you can take part.

# Glossary

A term in **bold** within an explanation indicates that it, too, is defined in this glossary.

**acute**  Short-lasting. In medical terms, this usually means lasting for days rather than weeks or months. (*See also* chronic)

**adrenal glands**  Important glands in the body that produce a number of hormones to control the body systems. Cortisol and cortisone are two very important examples, and adrenaline is another.

**allergens**  If you are allergic to something, allergens are the tiny particles or substances to which you react when you come into contact with them.

**allergy**  To have an allergy means to over-react to something in a harmful way when you come into contact with it. If you have an allergy to grass pollen you will have streaming eyes and nose and sneezing if you come into contact with it (hayfever). Someone who is not allergic to grass pollen will not even notice when they have come into contact with it.

**anaemia**  This means a reduction in the amount of the oxygen-carrying pigment, haemoglobin, in the blood.

**anaphylaxis**  An abnormal reaction to a particular **antigen**, which can lead to breathing problems, a skin rash, swelling and collapse.

**androgens**  These are **hormones** that stimulate the development of male sex organs and male secondary sexual characteristics (e.g. beard growth, deepening of the voice and muscle development). Very low levels are found in females.

**antibody**  A special kind of blood protein made in response to a particular **antigen,** which is designed to attack or neutralise the antigen.

**antigen**   Any substance that the body regards as foreign or potentially dangerous.

**antihistamine**   A drug that inhibits the action of histamine, which is one of the substances in the body involved in producing allergic reactions.

**atopic**   To be atopic is to have an inherited tendency to develop allergic or hypersensitive reactions. The three common atopic diseases are eczema, asthma and hayfever.

**atrophy**   Wasting away of a body tissue. With skin this means thinning and loss of strength.

**barrier cream**   A cream or ointment used to protect the skin against irritants.

**blister**   A swelling within the skin containing watery fluid and sometimes blood or pus.

**bone marrow**   The tissue contained within the internal cavities of bones that is involved in making blood cells.

**chronic**   In strictly medical terms, chronic means long-lasting or persistent. Many people use the word 'chronic' incorrectly to mean severe or extreme. (*See also* acute)

**dermatitis**   Another word for eczema, often used to imply that the cause is external rather than from within the body.

**dermatology**   The medical speciality concerned with the diagnosis and treatment of skin disease.

**dermis**   The deep layer of the skin.

**diagnostic**   Something that is 'diagnostic' occurs so often in a disease that you don't need any other clues to know what the disease is.

**dietician**   A specialist in nutrition.

**distribution**   The pattern of a disease on the skin; for example, all over, on the hands, in the flexures etc.

**eczema**   A red, itchy inflammation of the skin, sometimes with blisters and weeping.

**ELISA**   This stands for enzyme-linked immunosorbent assay; it is a sensitive technique to measure the amount of a substance in the blood by using **antibodies**.

**emollient**   An agent that soothes and softens the skin; also known as a moisturiser.

**emulsifying ointment**   A thick, greasy **emollient**.

**epidermis**   The outer layer of the skin.

**erythroderma**   An abnormal reddening, flaking and thickening of the skin, affecting a wide area of the body.

**extensor**   The side of a limb on which lie the muscles that straighten the limb (e.g. the back of the arm and the front of the leg).

**family therapist**   A psychologist who studies the way families interact and who tries to help with problems by clarifying and modifying this interaction.

**flexures**   The areas where the limbs bend, bringing two skin surfaces close together (e.g. the front of the elbow, the back of the knee and the groin).

**folliculitis**   An inflammation of the **hair follicles** in the skin.

**genes**   Units of inheritance that make up an individual's characteristics. Half are inherited from each parent.

**genetic**   To do with **genes**.

**hair follicles**   A specialised group of cells in the **dermis** that surround the root of a hair.

**health visitor**   A trained nurse with experience in midwifery and special training in preventive medicine and health education. Most of them deal with young children but some specialise in the care of the elderly.

**herpes virus**   One of the agents that can produce infections that can lie dormant in the body. Examples are herpes simplex causing cold sores, and herpes zoster causing chickenpox and shingles.

**hormone**   A substance that is produced in a gland in one part of the body and is carried in the bloodstream to work in other parts of the body.

**house dust mite**   A microscopic insect (Latin name *Dermatophagoides pteryonyssinus*). It survives by feeding on the dead scales of human skin that make up house dust.

**IgE**   Immunoglobulin E – one of a group of special proteins that act as **antibodies**.

**immune system**   The body's defence system against outside 'attackers' whether they are infections, injuries or agents that are recognised as 'foreign'. The immune system fights off infection and produces **antibodies** that will protect against future attack.

**immunity**   Resistance to specific disease(s) because of **antibodie** produced by the body's **immune system**.

**immunosuppressive**   A drug that reduces the body's resistance t infection and other foreign bodies by suppressing the immur reaction.

**in-patient therapy**   Treatment carried out when a patient admitted to hospital.

**incidence**   The number of new cases of an illness arising in population over a given time.

**inflammation**   The reaction of the body to an injury, infection ( disease. Generally, it will protect the body against the spread ( injury or infection, but may become **chronic**, when it tends damage the body rather than protect it.

**Interleukin-2**   One of a group of special proteins that control th immune response. Interleukin-2 stimulates the T-**lymphocyt** that are active in the skin.

**keratinocytes**   Types of cells that make up over 95% of th **epidermis** or outer layer of the skin.

**lichenification**   Thickening of the **epidermis**, with exaggeratic of the normal skin creases. The cause is excessive scratching ( rubbing of the skin.

**lymphocytes**   White blood cells that are involved in **immunity**

**malnutrition**   The condition resulting from an improper balan between what is eaten and what the body needs.

**moisturiser**   *See* emollient.

**natural history**   The normal course of a disease, the way develops over time.

**neurotransmitters**   Chemicals in the brain and nervous syste that relay electrical messages between nerve cells.

**paediatrician**   A specialist in diseases of childhood.

**papular**   A pattern of rash that consists of small raised spots ( the skin less than 5 mm in diameter.

**patch test**   A test to discover which **allergen** is responsible f contact **dermatitis**.

**pH**   The number reflects how acidic or alkaline a substance is: is neutral; a lower figure indicates acidic; a higher figure indicat alkaline.

**phototherapy**   Treatment with light – usually ultraviolet light

**placebo**   A medicine that is ineffective but may help to relieve condition because the patient has faith in its powers. New drugs are tested against placebos to make sure that they have a true active benefit in addition to the 'placebo response'.

**pompholyx**  A type of eczema on the hands and feet. Because the skin is so thick the tiny **blisters** do not rupture, so they persist in the skin – causing intense itching.

**psychologist**  A specialist who studies behaviour and its related mental processes.

**pustule**  A small pus-containing **blister**.

**rickets**  A disease of childhood in which the bones do not harden because of a deficiency of vitamin D.

**sebaceous glands**  Glands in the skin that produce an oily substance – sebum.

**seborrhoeic**  Related to excessive secretion of sebum (*see* sebaceous glands).

**skin-prick tests**  Special tests to show whether a person has a tendency to **allergy**. Drops of solution containing **allergen** are placed on the forearm and the skin is pricked through the solution. The result is 'positive' when a wheal, like a nettle rash, appears within 10 minutes. The tests are unreliable and carry a very small risk of a nasty reaction.

**steroids**  A particular group of chemicals, which includes very important **hormones**, produced naturally by the body, and also many drugs used for a wide range of medical purposes. In eczema the subgroup of steroids with which we are concerned is the corticosteroids. Very often this term is shortened to 'steroids', causing people to confuse their eczema treatments with the anabolic steroids used for body building.

**subcutaneous**  Beneath the skin.

**systemic**  This term is used for a drug given by mouth or injection that affects the whole body.

**triggers**  Factors that may bring on eczema but do not cause eczema.

**urticaria**  An itchy rash, looking like a nettle sting, caused by the release of histamine (*see also* antihistamine). Swellings on the skin appear rapidly and disappear within hours.

# APPENDIX 1

# Eczema associations and useful organisations

## ECZEMA AND SKIN CARE ASSOCIATIONS

National Eczema Society
163 Eversholt Street
London NW1 1BU
Tel: 0171-388 4097 (information staff available Mon to Fri, 9.30 a.m. to 5 p.m.)
Helpline: 0990 11 88 77 (24-hour information)
Website: www.eczema.org

The National Eczema Society was set up specifically to help people with eczema and those who look after them. A large proportion of the Society's members are parents whose children have eczema. Membership of the Society gives you access to:

- practical information and advice on all aspects of eczema and its treatment and management;
- the Society's full range of fact sheets and publications about eczema;
- support from the Society's nation-wide network of local contacts, all of whom have direct personal experience of eczema and the problems associated with it;
- the Society's highly respected quarterly magazine, *Exchange*.

In addition to the service it provides directly for people with eczema and their families, the Society runs eczema training courses for nurses (including health visitors), pharmacists and GPs. It encourages and sponsors research into the causes and treatment of eczema. And it campaigns to raise public awareness of eczema and to represent the interests of people with eczema.

Skin Care Campaign
163 Eversholt Street
London NW1 1BU
Tel: 0171-388 5651
Fax: 0171-388 5882

The Skin Care Campaign is an alliance of patient groups, companies and other organisations with a common interest in skin health. Administered by the National Eczema Society, it campaigns nationally to the government and to the NHS on behalf of skin patients. It campaigns through the media to raise awareness of skin issues among health professionals and the public at large. And it runs a series of popular Skin Information Days around the country and throughout the year.

## IN THE USA

National Eczema Association for Science and Education
1221 SW Yamhill
#303 Portland OR 97205
USA
Tel: 001 503 228 4430

An American association that produces a newsletter.

# ADVICE, HELP AND SUPPORT ON DISFIGUREMENT

Changing Faces
1–2 Junction Mews
London W2 1PN
Tel: 0171-706 4232
Fax: 0171-706 4234

Disfigurement Guidance Centre
PO Box 7
Cupar, Fife KY15 4PF
Tel: 01334 839084

Skinship (UK)
10 Thurstable Way
Tollesbury
Maldon, Essex CM9 8SQ
(please enclose s.a.e.)
Tel: 01621 868666

# HOLIDAYS

Peak (*formerly* Joint Holiday Project)
c/o National Asthma Campaign
Providence House
Providence Place
London N1 0NT
Tel: 0171-226 2260
Website: http://www.asthma.org.uk
Runs action-packed week-long holidays for children aged 6–17
years with asthma and/or eczema.
Website: http://www.asthma.org/Get_Involved/JHP/jhp.ntm

*IN THE USA*

Camp Horizon
Howard Pride MD
Department of Dermatology
Geisinger Medical Center
Danville PA 17822-1406
USA
A 'holiday project' in the USA for children aged 8–13 with
chronic skin diseases. Medically supervised and run by camp
counsellors who also have chronic skin disease.

# ORGANISATIONS FOR PROFESSIONALS

All Party Parliamentary Group on Skin
3/19 Holmbush Road
London SW15 3LE
Tel: 0181-789 2798
Fax: 0181-789 0795
An all-party group specialising in skin, which was established in
1993 to raise awareness in Parliament of skin disease.

British Association of Dermatologists
19 Fitzroy Square
London W1P 5HQ
Tel: 0171-383 0266
An association for dermatologists.

British Dermatology Nursing Group
19 Fitzroy Square
London W1P 5HQ
Tel: 0171-383 0266
A group, affiliated to the British Association of Dermatologists, that supports the growing numbers of specialist nurses working in dermatology.

British Skin Foundation
PO Box 6
Princes Risborough
Bucks HP27 9XD
Tel: 01844 347121
Fund raising for research.

Primary Care Dermatology Society
PO Box 6
Princes Risborough
Bucks HP27 9XD
Tel: 01844 347121
A society for GPs with a special interest in dermatology; also affiliated to the British Association of Dermatologists.

# APPENDIX 2

## *Other useful addresses*

Anaphylaxis Campaign
PO Box 149
Fleet
Hampshire GU13 9XU
Tel: 01252 542029
Fax: 01252 377140

Association of Breast Feeding Mothers
PO Box 207
Bridgwater
Somerset TA6 7YT
Tel: 0181-778 4769 (answerphone giving local contacts)
Fax: 0117-966 1788

British Allergy Foundation
Deepdene House
30 Belgrove Road
Welling, Kent DA16 3PY
Tel: 0181-303 8525
Fax 0181-303 8792
Helpline: 0891 516 500

British Homoeopathic Association
27a Devonshire Street
London W1N 1RJ
Tel: 0171-935 2163

Carers National Association
20–25 Glasshouse Yard
London EC1A 4JS
Tel: 0171-490 8818
Helpline: 0345 573369
(10 a.m.–noon and 2–4 p.m.)

Scotland:
3rd floor
162 Buchanan Street
Glasgow G1 2LL
Tel: 0141-333 9495

Supports all people who have to care for others because of medical or other problems.

DfEE Publications Centre
PO Box 5050
Sudbury
Suffolk CO10 6ZX
Tel: 0845-602 2260
Fax: 0845-603 3360

The Department for Education and Employment (DfEE) has produced a good-practice guide for schools, covering areas such as who is responsible for medication and policies for supporting pupils with medical needs. They also have a guide for parents on *Special Educational Needs*; copies are available in various languages.

Department of Social Security
Benefit Enquiry Line
Tel: 0800 882 200

Disability Alliance
1st floor East
Universal House
88–94 Wentworth Street
London E1 7SA
Tel: 0171-247 8776
Welfare rights enquiries: 0171-247 8763
(2–4 p.m., Mon and Wed)

Family Fund Trust
Information Officer
PO Box 50
York YO1 9ZX
Tel: 01904 621115
Textphone: 01904 658085
Helps families who care for severely disabled children under 16 by providing grants and information related to the care of the child.

Health Education Authority
Trevelyan House
30 Great Peter Street
London SW1P 2HW
Tel: 0171-222 5300
Orders: 01235 465 565
Promotion of, and publications and videos on, all aspects of general health (e.g. healthy eating, sensible drinking, stopping smoking, exercise).

National Asthma Campaign
Providence House
Providence Place
London N1 0NT
Tel: 0171-226 2260
Fax: 0171-704 0740
Website: http://www.asthma.org.uk

Research Council for Complementary Medicine
60 Great Ormond Street
London WC1N 3JF
Tel: 0171-833 8897

Society of Homoeopaths
2 Artisan Road
Northampton NN1 4HU
Tel: 01604 621400

# MAIL ORDER CLOTHING

Cotton Moon Ltd
Freepost (SE 8265)
PO Box 280
London SE3 8BR
Tel: 0181-305 0012

Schmidt Natural Clothing
21 Post Horn Close
Forest Row
East Sussex RH18 5DE
Tel/Fax: 01342 822169

The Silk Story
Freepost LON 7712
London SE16 4BR
Tel: 0171-231 9938

Vernon-Carus
Penwortham Mills
Preston
Lancs PR1 9SN
Tel: 01772 744493

# OTHER PRODUCTS

Eladon Limited
63 High Street
Bangor
Gwynedd LL57 1NR
Tel: 01248 370059
Suppliers of information and of herbal products that can be used
in eczema.

The National Eczema Society carries an up-to-date list of both
clothing companies and other companies that make products of
interest to people with eczema.

# APPENDIX 3

## Useful publications -

## GENERAL TITLES

*Eczema in Childhood: The facts* by David Atherton, published by Oxford University Press

*The Eczema Handbook* by Jenny Lewis, published by Vermilion

*Special Educational Needs: A guide for parents*, a booklet published by the Department for Education and Employment (see Appendix 2 for address)

*Sun Know How*, a catalogue by Louise Rees, published by Sun Know How, Health Education Authority, PO Box 269, Abingdon, Oxon OX14 4YN. Tel: 0171-222 5300

## BOOKS FOR PROFESSIONALS

*Atopic Skin Disease: A manual for practitioners* by Christopher Bridgett, Peter Noren and Richard Staughton, published by Wrighton Biomedical Publishing Ltd (1996)

## VIDEOS

*Live Without Eczema* by C Bridgett, available from the Medical Illustration Department, Chelsea and Westminster Hospital, London SW10 9NH (Ann McGarry: 0181-746 8262)

*Coping with Eczema* by J I Harper, available from Victoria Yates, Medical Illustration Department, Great Ormond Street Children's Fund, Hospital for Sick Children, Great Ormond Street, 40–41 Queen Square, London WC1N 3AJ

*Emergency! Coping with medical crises in school,* a BBC video covering asthma, eczema and epilepsy in the classroom, available from BBC Educational Publishing, PO Box 234, Wetherby, W Yorks LS23 7EU (Credit card sales tel: 01937 541001, 9 a.m.–4 p.m.)

# Index

Have you found **Eczema and your child: a parent's guide** practical and useful? If so, you may be interested in other books from Class Publishing.

## Allergies at your fingertips
NEW! £11.95
*Dr Joanne Clough*

At last – sensible practical advice on allergies from an experienced medical expert.

> 'Extremely enjoyable and informative.'
> *Susan Ollier BSc, Scientific Director, British Allergy Foundation*

## Skin care for psoriasis £7.95
*Dr V K Dave*

This book shows you how to control your psoriasis and teaches you self-help measures for looking after your skin.

> Easy to follow, practical help guide.'
> *Prof. Griffiths, Professor of Dermatology, University of Manchester*

## Find your way around the NHS
£9.95
*Dr Jo Clough and Dr Alan Glasper*

This essential guide from two medical practitioners will help you make sense of any visit to your doctor or hospital. The book tells you what to expect – and also what you are entitled to.

## High blood pressure at your fingertips £11.95
*Dr Julian Tudor Hart*

The author uses all his 26 years of experience as a General Practitioner and blood pressure expert to answer your questions on high blood pressure.

> 'Readable and comprehensive information.'
> *Dr Sylvia McLaughlan, Director General, The Stroke Association*

## Asthma at your fingertips
NEW SECOND EDITION
£11.95
*Dr Mark Levy,
Professor Sean Hilton and
Greta Barnes MBE*

This book shows you how to keep your asthma – or your family's asthma – under control, making it easier to live a full, happy and healthy life.

> 'This book gives you the knowledge. Don't limit yourself.'
> *Adrian Moorhouse MBE, Olympic Gold Medallist*

## Stop that heart attack!
NEW! £14.99
*Dr Derrick Cutting*

The easy, drug-free and medically *accurate* way to cut dramatically your risk of suffering a heart attack.

Even if you already have heart disease, you can halt or even reverse its progress by following Dr Cutting's simple steps. Don't be a victim – take action now!

## Heart health at your fingertips
NEW! £14.95
*Dr Graham Jackson*

Everything you need to know to keep your heart healthy – and live life to the full! This practical handbook, written by a leading cardiologist, answers all your questions about heart conditions – from diagnosis to treatment, and from work to relationships.

## Diabetes at your fingertips
NEW FOURTH EDITION
£14.95
*Professor Peter Sonksen,*
*Dr Charles Fox and*
*Sister Sue Judd*

461 questions on diabetes are answered clearly and accurately – the ideal reference book for everyone with diabetes.
> 'I will certainly recommend it to my patients ... I think it is brilliant.'
> *Robert Tattersall, Professor of Clinical Diabetes, Queen's Medical Centre, Nottingham*

## Parkinson's at your fingertips
£11.95
*Dr Marie Oxtoby and*
*Professor Adrian Williams*

Full of practical help and advice for people with Parkinson's disease and their families. This book gives you the information and the confidence to tackle the challenges that PD presents.
> 'A super DIY manual for patients and carers.'
> *Dr Bernard Dean*

## Epilepsy at your fingertips
NEW! £14.95
*Brian Chappell and*
*Dr Pamela Crawford*

All your questions about epilepsy and how to manage it are answered in plain English by the two expert authors. If you – or anyone in your family – has epilepsy, you will find this practical handbook invaluable.

## Alzheimer's at your fingertips
NEW! £11.95
*Harry Cayton, Dr Nori Graham and Dr James Warner*

At last – a book that tells you everything you need to know about Alzheimer's and other dementias.
> 'An invaluable contribution to understanding all forms of dementia.'
> *Dr Jonathan Miller, CBE, President of the Alzheimer's Disease Society*

## Cancer information at your fingertips
NEW SECOND EDITION
£11.95
*Val Speechley and*
*Maxine Rosenfield*

Recommended by the Cancer Research Campaign, this book provides straightforward, practical and positive answers to all your questions about cancer.

## Epilepsy and your child: a parent's guide £9.95
*Dr Richard Appleton,*
*Brian Chappell and*
*Sister Margaret Beirne*

Epilepsy is a baffling subject to be faced with. This practical handbook answers real questions asked by parents of children with epilepsy.
 Their experience and the authors' expert answers give you the knowledge to help your child lead a happy, healthy and normal life.

# PRIORITY ORDER FORM

Cut out or photocopy this form and send it (post free in the UK) to:

Class Publishing Priority Service
FREEPOST (no stamp needed)
London W6 7BR

Tel: 01752 202301

Fax: 01752 202333

Please send me urgently
(tick boxes below)

**Post included
price per copy
(UK only)**

| |  |  |
|---|---|---|
| ☐ | **Eczema and your child: a parent's guide** (ISBN 1 872362 86 9) | £14.95 |
| ☐ | **Allergies at your fingertips** (ISBN 1 872362 52 4) | £14.95 |
| ☐ | **Skin care for psoriasis** (ISBN 1 872362 63 X) | £10.95 |
| ☐ | **Find your way around the NHS** (ISBN 1 872362 75 3) | £12.95 |
| ☐ | **High blood pressure at your fingertips** (ISBN 1 872362 48 6) | £14.95 |
| ☐ | **Asthma at your fingertips** (ISBN 1 872362 67 2) | £14.95 |
| ☐ | **Stop that heart attack!** (ISBN 1 872362 85 0) | £17.99 |
| ☐ | **Heart health at your fingertips** (ISBN 1 872362 77 X) | £17.95 |
| ☐ | **Diabetes at your fingertips** (ISBN 1 872362 79 6) | £17.95 |
| ☐ | **Parkinson's at your fingertips** (ISBN 1 872362 47 8) | £14.95 |
| ☐ | **Epilepsy at your fingertips** (ISBN 1 872362 51 6) | £17.95 |
| ☐ | **Alzheimer's at your fingertips** (ISBN 1 872362 71 0) | £14.95 |
| ☐ | **Cancer information at your fingertips** (ISBN 1 872362 56 7) | £14.95 |
| ☐ | **Epilepsy and your child: a parent's guide** (ISBN 1 872362 61 3) | £12.95 |

TOTAL: _____

**Easy ways to pay**

Cheque: I enclose a cheque payable to Class Publishing for £_____

Credit card: Please debit my ☐ Access ☐ Visa ☐ Amex ☐ Switch

Number: _____ Expiry date: _____

Name _____

My address for delivery is _____

_____

Town _____ County _____ Postcode _____

Telephone number (in case of query) _____

Credit card billing address if different from above _____

_____

Town _____ County _____ Postcode _____

Class Publishing's guarantee: remember that if, for any reason, you are not satisfied with these books, we will refund all your money, without any questions asked. Prices and VAT rates may be altered for reasons beyond our control.